HEALTHCARE LIBRAR

The North Hampshire H

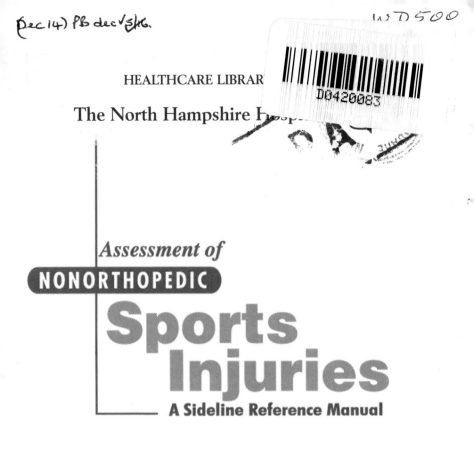

Assessment of

NONORTHOPEDIC

Sports
Injuries

A Sideline Reference Manual

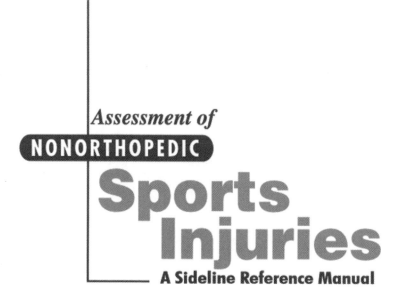

Assessment of
NONORTHOPEDIC
Sports
Injuries
A Sideline Reference Manual

JEFFREY LEWANDOWSKI, DPT, SCS, ATC

PHYSICAL THERAPIST AND ADMINISTRATOR
HEALTHSOUTH SPORTS MEDICINE AND REHABILITATION CENTER
KENNESAW, GEORGIA

CLINICAL FACULTY
EMORY UNIVERSITY MEDICAL SCHOOL
DEPARTMENT OF PHYSICAL MEDICINE AND REHABILITATION
DIVISION OF PHYSICAL THERAPY
ATLANTA, GEORGIA

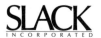

SLACK
INCORPORATED

6900 Grove Road • Thorofare, NJ 08086

Publisher: John H. Bond
Editorial Director: Amy E. Drummond

Lewandowski, Jeffrey.
    Assessment of nonorthopedic sports injuries: a sideline reference manual/Jeffrey Lewandowski.
        p.;cm.
    Includes bibliographical references and index.
    ISBN 1-55642-444-2 (alk. paper)
    1. Sports injuries—Diagnosis—Handbooks, manuals, etc. I. Title.
    [DNLM: 1. Athletic injuries—diagnosis—Handbooks. QT 29 L669e 2000]
    RD97.L49 2000
    617.1'027-dc21   99-086957

Printed in the United States of America.
Published by: SLACK Incorporated
                6900 Grove Road
                Thorofare, NJ 08086-9447 USA
                Telephone: 856-848-1000
                Fax: 856-853-5991
                www.slackinc.com

Contact SLACK Incorporated for more information about other books in this field or about the availability of our books from distributors outside the United States.

Last digit is print number: 10 9 8 7 6 5 4 3 2 1

DEDICATION

To my parents, Elaine and Rich, for all their love, guidance, and support.

CONTENTS

ACKNOWLEDGMENTS

I would like to thank the following people for their help in writing this manual: my doctoral committee members, including Robert Kelly, MD; Peter Loubert, PhD, PT, ATC; and M. Shay Womack, MD, for their guidance and assistance; all of my colleagues and students for their suggestions and editing assistance.

About the Author

Jeffrey Lewandowski, DPT, SCS, ATC received his undergraduate degree in exercise science from the University of Missouri, Columbia; his physical therapy degree from Rockhurst College, Kansas City, Mo; and his Master of Science degree in exercise science from Georgia State University, Atlanta. While attending Georgia State, he worked in the training room at the Georgia Institute of Technology, where he gained valuable information on the evaluation and treatment of athletic injuries. Dr. Lewandowski received an advanced clinical doctorate degree in physical therapy, specializing in sport medicine, from the University of St. Augustine for Health Sciences, St. Augustine, Fla.

Dr Lewandowski is a board certified sports physical therapist and a certified athletic trainer. Throughout his 14 years of clincal experience, Dr. Lewandowski has had the opportunity to provide sports medicine coverage and treatment for athletes at the high school, college, amature, and professional levels. He is currently a practicing physical therapist and administrator with Healthsouth Corporation in Atlanta, Ga. He is also currently on the clincal faculty staff at Emory University in Atlanta.

PREFACE

This project was completed in partial fulfillment for the requirements of attaining an advanced clinical doctorate degree in physical therapy from the University of St. Augustine for Health Sciences. This book is designed to be used by sports medicine clinicians and students. It is meant to be a quick and user-friendly reference guide to help the clinician evaluate and treat nonorthopedic injuries. Most sports medicine clinicians are well experienced in orthopedics and can usually evaluate and treat orthopedic sports injuries with relative ease. However, when faced with a nonorthopedic injury, the clinician may have difficulty remembering the specific evaluation techniques and assessments, important signs and symptoms, and the initial treatment of the injury. Therefore, this book is designed to be a useful tool to the clinician, especially when performing a secondary evaluation. It will also be useful as a supplemental learning text for the sports medicine student who has knowledge in anatomy. This book is not intended for use by a lay person or coach.

Users of this book should keep several things in mind. First, the chapters follow the same format. The chapters begin with an introduction, followed by an algorithm, tables that highlight the algorithm, a brief anatomy review (when needed), and tables that briefly describe specific pathological processes. Second, the algorithms are fairly comprehensive. Therefore, it is strongly recommended that the user review the book before using it on the sidelines. Third, the book is designed for quick referencing. The tabs in the book assist the clinician by allowing him or her to quickly locate a specific evaluation algorithm. Also, nodes in the algorithms that involve an evaluative action to be taken by the clinician are shaded in gray for quicker reference. Additionally, medical terminology is defined within the body of the pages. The algorithms follow a specific pattern. They are designed to first rule out any potentially catastrophic injuries, such as cervical spine and head injuries. The algorithms then guide the clinician through an evaluation specific to the context of the chapter. As the algorithms progress through the evaluation, they differentiate between the signs and symptoms that are indicative of serious conditions from those that are relatively benign. Thus, the algorithm evaluations are not designed to diagnose injuries, but to screen out potential conditions that require further medical evaluation and treatment. When in doubt of your evaluation findings and assessment, err on the side of conservatism and refer the injured athlete for further medical evaluation.

—Jeffrey Lewandowski, DPT, SCS, ATC

CHAPTER 1

Initial Evaluation of the Injured Athlete

The purpose of this chapter is to the give the reader a general overview and introduction to the evaluation of an injured athlete. It includes reference material that is referred to in the rest of the chapters, such as normal vital sign parameters, how to activate the emergency medical service (EMS), and performing a rapid body assessment. Therefore, this chapter is not intended to be used alone when performing an evaluation of an injured athlete on the field. It is also to be used to augment the material in the other chapters that deal with the evaluation of specific injuries.

Although most sports injuries are minor in nature, catastrophic injuries do occur. It is important to be prepared for such emergencies.[1,2] All sports medicine clinicians and coaches should have an emergency plan in place that covers all practices and games. This includes several factors. First, access to a phone is required at all times. Instructions for EMS activation should be written down and placed near the phone. Second, emergency vehicles must have access to the practice and playing fields. Third, emergency supplies need to be placed at all potential sites of injury. Fourth, each individual needs to have a defined role in the event of an emergency. Different individuals need to be specifically responsible to initially evaluate the athlete, place the EMS call, bring needed emergency supplies to the evaluating clinician, and meet the emergency vehicle at the entrance/gate in order to direct it to the location of the injured athlete.

When evaluating a potentially serious injury, several steps should be followed. The first is to recognize that an injury has occurred. When providing sports medicine coverage, it is important for the clinician to remain alert at all times. The clinician must observe all of the athletes on the field of play. The clinician needs to avoid concentrating only on the center of action in a game or practice. Second, when approaching an injured athlete, assess the safety of the scene, mechanism of injury, need for assistance, and the possible need for cervical spine and/or universal precautions.[1,2] Third, it is important to initially evaluate the athlete as soon as possible and, whenever possible, at the scene of the injury.[3,4] If the athlete is moved too quickly before a thorough initial evaluation is performed, an unstable condition (eg, cervical spine fracture) can develop into a catastrophic injury. Also, it is important to document the time of the injury and when evaluative findings were found (ie, time that the pulse, blood pressure, etc were taken). Due to emotional stress, a clinician can at times become confused and even forgetful when evaluating an athlete with a potentially serious injury. Therefore, the fourth step is for the clinician to adopt and follow a consistent systematic approach to all evaluations. The clinician also needs to keep calm and take the time to perform a complete evaluation. Do not feel rushed by coaches, officials, fans, or the injured athlete.[3] Be sure to screen for hidden injuries, especially in the presence of an obvious injury.[4] For example, if an athlete injures an eye due to a blow to the orbital region, make sure that he or she does not also have an underlying cervical or head injury. Make sure to document all results and findings.

After the initial evaluation, a decision must be made to initiate the EMS, hold the athlete out of play and refer him or her to a physician, or decide that no significant injury has occurred and allow the athlete return to play. If no injury is initially apparent, continue to re-evaluate the athlete over minutes, hours, or days as needed, in order to make a complete assessment. This is especially important in the case of a head, abdominal, or thoracic injury. Promptly refer the injured athlete to a physician if you are unsure of the evaluation findings, assessment, or treatment. Remember the "Golden Hour": A critically injured patient (danger of death) needs physician/medical care and/or surgery within 1 hour of the injury in order to have the best chance for a favorable outcome.[5]

GENERAL EVALUATION OF AN INJURED ATHLETE

Apparent Injury

EMS: Emergency Medical Service.
PRN: As Needed.
CPR: Cardiopulmonary Resuscitation.

Ask the Athlete:
"Where are you hurt?"
or
"Are you OK?"

Verbally Unresponsive

Verbally Responsive

Stabilize Cervical Spine

Abnormal → Evaluate **A**, **B**, **C**, **D**'s (Tables 1-2, 1-3)

Normal

Assess the following:
- **A**irway (Table 1-1)-Open, Partial or Complete Obstruction.
- **B**reathing (Table 1-2)-Rate, Quality.
- **C**irculation (Table 1-2)-Pulse, Rate, Rhythm, Strength.
- **D**ysfunction (Table 1-3)-AVPU.

Rule Out Cervical Spine Injury:
1. Questions:
- Neck pain
- Extremity Paralysis.
- Extremity Movement and Strength.
2. Cervical Spine Palpation.

Abnormal

Normal

Is the Athlete Breathing?
and
Is There a Pulse?

No   Yes

Chief Complaint
SAMPLE History (Table 1-5)
Vital Signs (Table 1-2):
- Pulse.
- Respirations.
- Pupils.
- Temperature.
- Skin Color.
- Mental Status (Table 1-6).
- Level of Consciousness (Table 1-7).
- Rapid Assessment (Table 1-8).

Abnormal

Activate EMS (Table 1-4)

Stabilize Cervical Spine

Initiate CPR

Normal

- Systemic Abnormality.
- Visceral Abnormality.
- Gross Orthopedic Instability.

Abnormal

Focused Exam
- Orthopedic and/or
- Non Orthopedic (see specific chapters)

Non-Emergent Dysfunction Identified

No Identified Dysfunctions Present

Activate EMS (Table 1-4).
Access Airway.
Monitor A, B, C, D's (Tables 1-2, 1-3).
Monitor Vital Signs (Table 1-2).
Rapid Body Assessment (Table 1-8).
Control Bleeding PRN.
Supportive Care.
Stabilize Body Part (if Unstable Musculoskeletal Dysfunction).

PRN   Physician Referral PRN

Return to Play

PRN

Treatment by Sports Physical Therapist/Certified Athletic Trainer PRN

Table 1-1

Airway

Obstructions:
- Tongue: most common
- Objects: foreign body, teeth, vomitus, blood
- Throat swelling: allergic reaction, trauma

Methods to Open Airway:
- Head tilt and chin lift
- Jaw thrust if suspect cervical spine injury

Table 1-2

Vital Signs

Sign	Normal	Abnormality	Interpretation
Breathing[4,5]—rates	Adult: 12 breaths/min Child: 20 to 25 breaths/min	Tachypnea (rapid breathing) > 24	
	Conditioned athlete: 6 to 8 breaths/min	1. Rapid and shallow 2. Rapid and deep Dyspnea (shortness of breath) < 8 breaths/min; deep, labored and noisy gasping	1. Shock 2. Severe head injury Partial airway obstruction or respiratory failure
Breathing—noises	Quiet	Snoring	Partial airway obstruction
		Stridor/crowing Wheezing	Laryngeal obstruction Lower airway obstruction; asthma
		Gurgling	Fluid
Breathing—rhythms	Effortless and cyclical	Central neurogenic hyperventilation (rapid deep pattern)	Hyperventilation; head injury; extreme exertion
		Kussmaul respirations (deep and gasping)	Diabetic coma
		Cheyne-Stokes pattern (increasing and decreasing rate and volume)	Head injury
		Biot's respiration (irregular pattern of apnea and hyperventilation)	Head injury
Pulse[1,3-7]	Adult: 60 to 80 beats/min Child: 80 to 100 beats/min	Rapid and weak	Shock; heat exhaustion; hemorrhage; diabetic coma
	Conditioned athlete: 45 to 60 beats/min	Rapid and strong Slow and strong Bounding (pulse appears to be strong and bouncing but somewhat normal in rate)	Heat stroke; fright Head injury; stroke High blood pressure; fright
		Irregular Drop > 15 to 20 beats/min in standing vs lying	Cardiac dysrhythmia Orthostatic hypotension (a drop in blood pressure when going from a reclined to an upright position)

Table 1-2, continued

Sign	Normal	Abnormality	Interpretation
Blood pressure[4,5]	Male systolic: 100+ age, up to 140 to 150 mmHg	Low blood pressure	Shock; heat illness; internal organ injury
	Male diastolic: 60 to 90 mmHg	Increasing systolic with same or decreasing diastolic	Head injury
	Female: 10 mmHg lower than males	Decreasing systolic with possible increasing diastolic	Tension pneumothorax; cardiac tamponade
Pupils[5]	Consensual (together), quick reaction to light	Dilation	Unconsciousness; pain; decreased blood oxygen; head injury; shock; CNS* stimulant medication; cardiac arrest
		Constriction	CNS depressant medication
		Slow reacting	Hypoxia (decreased blood oxygen); hypercarbia (increased blood carbon dioxide); CNS depressant medication; general injury
		Anisocoria (pupil inequality)	Head injury; stroke; normal response in some individuals
		Doll's eye response (eyes move with the head during rotation)	Head injury
Temperature (indicative of circulation and/or core temp)	Normal core: 98.6°F or 37°C	Cool and clammy	Trauma; shock; heat exhaustion
	Normal skin: neutral and dry; hot and sweaty during exercise	Cool and dry	Hypothermia
		Hot and dry	Disease; infection; fever; heat stroke
Skin color[3-6] (indicative of circulation and/or level of blood oxygen)	Pink or tan in white athletes	Abnormal for white athletes: Red (increased blood circulation)	Heat stroke; high blood pressure; fever; poisoning; alcohol ingestion
	Note: capillary refill for athletes of all color should be 2 seconds or less.	Pale/white (decreased circulation)	Shock; hemorrhage; heat exhaustion; insulin shock; fright; cold exposure
	Dark pigmented athletes: nail beds, mucous membranes of eyes, and tissues under the tongue should be pink	Abnormal for dark pigmented athletes: gray cast around nose and mouth and/or bluish nail beds and mucous membranes	Shock
		Pale, gray, waxy membranes of mouth and tongue	Hypovolemia (decreased intravascular volume)

*CNS=central nervous system

Table 1-3

Dysfunction (of Consciousness)[3]

A—Alert: Aware (to person, time, and place) and responds appropriately and quickly to questions asked.
V—Verbal: Not alert, but responds to verbal commands.
P—Pain: Only responds to pain (pinch thumb web space or rub knuckles on sternum).
U—Unresponsive.

Table 1-4

EMS Phone Call[1,3,5,6]

- Location of emergency
- Name and phone number of caller
- Number of injured athletes and their conditions
- What happened/mechanism of injury
- Treatment rendered to the injured athlete
- Specific directions to location, including landmarks
- Any other information needed
- Let the EMS operator hang up first

Table 1-5

SAMPLE History[2,5]

S—Symptoms: provocation, quality, region, severity, timing (PQRST)
A—Allergies
M—Medications: Over-the-counter, prescribed, or illegal drugs or performance-enhancing substances
P—Past medical history
L—Last meal consumed
E—Events preceding the injury (ie, mechanism of injury)

Table 1-6

Mental Status

- Person: What is your name?
- Place: Where are you?
- Time: What is the day or date? How old are you?
- Retrograde amnesia: What events led up to the injury?
- Anterograde amnesia: What do you first recall after the injury?

Table 1-7

Level of Consciousness (Glasgow Scale)

Eye Opening	Spontaneous	4
	To voice	3
	To pain	2
	None	1
Motor Response	Obeys commands	6
	Purposeful movement	5
	Withdraws to pain	4
	Flexion posturing	3
	Extension posturing	2
	None	1
Verbal Response	Oriented	5
	Confused	4
	Inappropriate words	3
	Incomprehensible sounds	2
	None	1
Possible Score		3 to 15

Table 1-8
Rapid Body Assessment[5]

Head (Cranium, Face, Ears)
- Visual inspection
- Palpation for asymmetries or crepitation
- Pupils
- Inspect for fluid in ears, nose, and mouth:
  - Presence of blood or cerebral spinal fluid (clear): fracture or laceration
  - Halo test: collect nasal drainage with a clean gauze pad. If there is a red dot (blood) surrounded by a ring of clear fluid, suspect a cerebrospinal fluid leak
- Mouth odors:
  - Alcohol: consider intoxication
  - Ketones/fruity smell: diabetic coma
  - Fecal odor: lower bowel obstruction
  - Gastric odor: forewarning of vomitus

Neck
- Visual inspection and palpation
- Assess for jugular vein distention (JVD):
  - In an upright position, no JVD should be present
  - Below 45 degrees of body inclination with the head elevated (ie, in supine), mild JVD normally occurs
  - Abnormal increase in JVD (when upright): tension pneumothorax (air leak in the pleural space that causes lung to collapse and press against the heart and contralateral lung), pericardial tamponade (accumulation of fluid between the pericardium and the heart), corpulmonal (right congestive heart failure due to increased pulmonary resistance)
  - No JVD in supine: hypovolemia
- Assess for tracheal deviation during inspiration:
  - Contralateral deviation occurs with a tension pneumothorax
  - Ipsilateral deviation occurs with a simple pneumothorax or airway obstruction

Chest
- Visual inspection and palpation for deformity, symmetrical excursion with respiration, and respiration patterns
- Auscultation (listening with a stethoscope), if trained/experienced

Abdomen and Pelvis
- Visual inspection
- Palpation of all four quadrants
- Assess genitalia PRN

Assess Extremities
- Brief orthopedic evaluation
- PMS (pulse, motor, sensation)

Assess Posterior Trunk

References

1. Athletic Training Emergency Care. *Course Notebook*. Wichita, Kan, April 1997 (c/o DCH Outpatient Services, 809 University Boulevard East, Tuscaloosa, AL 35401).
2. Nowlan W, Davis G, McDonald B. Preparing for sudden emergencies. *Athletic Therapy Today*. 1996;1(1):45-47.
3. Booher J, Thibodeau G. *Athletic Injury Assessment. 3rd ed*. St. Louis, Mo: Mosby; 1994:196-289.
4. Voight M. Emergency care and on-the-field management. In: Sanders B, ed. *Sports Physical Therapy*. Norwalk, Conn: Appleton & Lange; 1990:45-59.
5. Bledsoe B, Porter R, Shade B. *Brady Paramedic Emergency Care. 3rd ed*. Upper Saddle River, NJ: Brady Prentice Hall; 1997:165-203.
6. Arnheim D. *Modern Principles of Athletic Training*. St. Louis, Mo: Times Mirror/Mosby College Publishing; 1989:248-297.
7. Halpern B. Injuries and emergencies on the field. In: Mellion M, Walsh W, Shelton G, eds. *The Team Physician's Handbook*. Philadelphia, Pa: Hanley & Belfus; 1990:128-142.

Bibliography

Marder R. On-field emergencies. In: Scuderi G, McCann P, Bruno P, eds. *Sports Medicine: Principles of Primary Care*. St. Louis, Mo: Mosby; 1996:74-85.

CHAPTER 2

Syncope and Near Syncope
(Transient Loss of Consciousness)

Syncope is a transient loss of consciousness (TLOC) and muscle tone. Prodromal symptoms are symptoms that an individual may experience just prior to a syncopal episode. This is also referred to as near syncope. It is possible to have prodromal symptoms (near syncope) without progressing to a TLOC (syncope). For example, an athlete may present with symptoms of feeling dizzy and light-headed but not lose consciousness. Also, if an athlete presents with near syncope and is treated properly, syncope may be avoided. The two basic forms of syncope (and near syncope) are cardiovascular and noncardiovascular.

The purpose of this chapter is to help the clinician assess benign forms of syncope from those that are more serious in nature. Syncope can be benign (orthostatic hypotension, vasovagal reactions, hyperventilation, mild hypoglycemia, and asthma attacks) which, in most cases, can be treated by the PT/ATC. Cardiogenic syncope and all other noncardiovascular syncope are more serious in nature, can be potentially life-threatening, and require medical referral. In general, the causes of syncope are as follows: 25% cardiogenic, 25% vasovagal, 10% to 25% miscellaneous disorders, and 25% to 40% idiopathic.[1] The most common causes of syncope in athletes are medications, drug use, hypovolemia, and vasovagal reactions.[2]

Cardiovascular syncope is caused by a decrease in cerebral blood flow. The three types of cardiovascular syncope are cardiogenic, orthostatic hypotension, and vasovagal reactions.[1,3,4] Cardiogenic syncope is due to mechanical or electrical changes in the heart that lead to a decrease in cardiac output, with a secondary decrease in cerebral blood flow. Orthostatic hypotension is a decrease in blood pressure when changing from a reclined to an elevated position. Hypovolemia is a decrease in intravascular volume and is a form of orthostatic hypotension. A vasovagal reaction is caused by stimulation of the vagus nerve/parasympathetic nervous system that causes a decrease in blood pressure and heart rate, leading to a decrease in cerebral blood flow. In cardiovascular syncope, most occurrences happen when the athlete is in the standing position. Also, there is usually a rapid return of mental status after consciousness is regained.[5,6]

Noncardiovascular syncope is caused by neurogenic, metabolic, anaphylactic reaction, heat stroke, or psychiatric disorders.[1,3,4] In noncardiovascular syncope, a syncope attack can occur in any position (upright, sitting, or lying). Also, there usually is not a rapid return of mental status after consciousness is returned.[5,6]

In many cases of syncope, a detailed history and assessment of vital signs can be most helpful in determining the cause.[4,7] When evaluating an athlete with syncope, keep in mind that in severe syncope episodes, secondary urinary incontinence and seizures may occur.[1,5,8] Therefore, it can be easy to mistake syncope for a frank seizure. A frank seizure must first be ruled out when evaluating syncope.[1,5,8] Seizures can be caused by many underlying cerebral conditions. Like noncardiovascular syncope, seizures can occur in any postural position. When trying to differentiate syncope from a seizure, the clinician should be aware that seizures are usually preceded by an aura (hallucinations, illusions, odor sensations, cognitive and affective changes). The clinician must be careful in order to differentiate auras from prodromal symptoms. Grand mal seizures are most easily misdiagnosed as syncope.

Evaluation of Syncope and/or Faintness

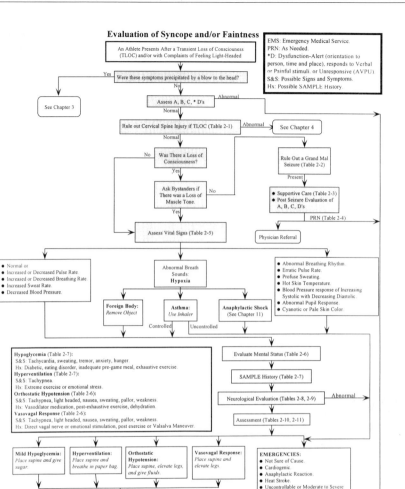

EMS: Emergency Medical Service.
PRN: As Needed.
*D: Dysfunction-Alert (orientation to person, time and place), responds to Verbal or Painful stimuli, or Unresponsive (AVPU).
S&S: Possible Signs and Symptoms.
Hx: Possible SAMPLE History.

An Athlete Presents After a Transient Loss of Consciousness (TLOC) and/or with Complaints of Feeling Light-Headed

Were these symptoms precipitated by a blow to the head? — Yes → See Chapter 3

No → Assess A, B, C, *D's — Abnormal → See Chapter 4

Normal → Rule out Cervical Spine Injury if TLOC (Table 2-1) — Abnormal →

Normal → Was There a Loss of Consciousness? — No →

Yes → Ask Bystanders if There was a Loss of Muscle Tone. — No →

Rule Out a Grand Mal Seizure (Table 2-2)

Present →
● Supportive Care (Table 2-3)
● Post Seizure Evaluation of A, B, C, D's

PRN (Table 2-4)

Physician Referral

Yes → Assess Vital Signs (Table 2-5)

● Normal or
● Increased or Decreased Pulse Rate.
● Increased or Decreased Breathing Rate.
● Increased Sweat Rate.
● Decreased Blood Pressure.

Abnormal Breath Sounds **Hypoxia**

● Abnormal Breathing Rhythm.
● Erratic Pulse Rate.
● Profuse Sweating.
● Hot Skin Temperature.
● Blood Pressure response of Increasing Systolic with Decreasing Diastolic.
● Abnormal Pupil Response.
● Cyanotic or Pale Skin Color.

Foreign Body: *Remove Object*

Asthma: *Use Inhaler* — Controlled / Uncontrolled

Anaphylactic Shock (See Chapter 11)

Hypoglycemia (Table 2-7):
S&S: Tachycardia, sweating, tremor, anxiety, hunger.
Hx: Diabetic, eating disorder, inadequate pre-game meal, exhaustive exercise.
Hyperventilation (Table 2-7):
S&S: Tachypnea.
Hx: Extreme exercise or emotional stress.
Orthostatic Hypotension (Table 2-6):
S&S: Tachypnea, light headed, nausea, sweating, pallor, weakness.
Hx: Vasodilator medication, post-exhaustive exercise, dehydration.
Vasovagal Response (Table 2-6):
S&S: Tachypnea, light headed, nausea, sweating, pallor, weakness.
Hx: Direct vagal nerve or emotional stimulation, post exercise or Valsalva Maneuver.

Evaluate Mental Status (Table 2-6)

SAMPLE History (Table 2-7)

Neurological Evaluation (Tables 2-8, 2-9) — Abnormal →

Assessment (Tables 2-10, 2-11)

Mild Hypoglycemia: *Place supine and give sugar.*

Hyperventilation: *Place supine and breathe in paper bag.*

Orthostatic Hypotension: *Place supine, elevate legs, and give fluids.*

Vasovagal Response: *Place supine and elevate legs.*

EMERGENCIES:
● Not Sure of Cause.
● Cardiogenic.
● Anaphylactic Reaction.
● Heat Stroke.
● Uncontrollable or Moderate to Severe Bleeding.
● All Other Non Cardiovascular causes.

Continue to Reassess for 30 Minutes
● Vital Signs.
● Mental Status.
● Signs and Symptoms.

Abnormal →

Normal → Return to Play if No Signs or Symptoms are Present for 30 Minutes (preferably with physician clearance).

Activate EMS
Stabilize Cervical Spine PRN
Monitor ABCD's
Monitor Vital Signs
Rapid Body Assessment PRN
Control Bleeding PRN
Supportive Care

Table 2-1

Some Signs and Symptoms of a Significant Cervical Spine Injury[9,10]

- Involuntary loss of bowel and/or bladder control
- Cervical pain without movement
- Pain with palpation over the posterior or anterior cervical spine
- Rigid muscle spasms of the anterior and/or posterior neck muscles
- Deformity detected by palpation or the presence of a wryneck (abnormal neck position usually including flexion, rotation, and side-bending)
- Decreased cervical spine mobility with pain
- Persistent burning, weakness, tingling, or numbness in any extremity

Table 2-2

Phases of Grand Mal Seizures[8]

- First phase: Flexing and abducting arms while extending legs
- Tonic phase: Vocalization, closure of mouth, incontinence
- Clonic phase: Violent muscle contractions, facial grimacing, respiratory apnea
- Seizures last 1 to 5 minutes
- Postseizure symptoms last 30 minutes to several hours: Confusion, drowsiness, fatigue, and headaches

Table 2-3

Supportive Care During a Seizure[3,9]

- Assist the athlete to the ground
- Clear the area of dangerous objects that the athlete may strike
- Never put objects or your fingers in the athlete's mouth
- Evaluate the A, B, C, and Ds after the seizure has stopped

Table 2-4

Some Signs and Symptoms of a Seizure that Require Immediate Medical Referral

- Compromised breathing
- The need for CPR
- Several seizures occur in a row without a return to baseline
- Mental confusion that lasts longer than 30 minutes
- This is the athlete's first seizure

Make an immediate medical referral when in doubt regarding the seriousness of the injury.

Table 2-5

Vital Signs—Possible Abnormal Findings in the Presence of Syncope*

Vital Sign	Abnormality	Interpretation
Pulse	Rapid rate	Hypoglycemia; hypovolemia; hypoxia; heat illness; pulmonary embolism; fever; drug toxicity
	Slow rate	Vasovagal reaction; cerebral injuries; hypokalemia
	Erratic rate	Cardiac dysfunction
	Decrease >15 to 20 beats/min in standing vs supine	Orthostatic hypotension
Blood pressure	Increasing systolic with same or decreasing diastolic	Head injury
	Decreased	Orthostatic hypotension; pulmonary embolism; heat stroke; anaphylactic reaction
Respiration	Increased rate	Heat illness; hypoxia; pulmonary embolism; hyperventilation
	Decreased rate	Heat stroke; pulmonary embolism; pneumothorax
	Abnormal sounds	Hypoxia
	Abnormal rhythm	Head injury
Skin temperature and moisture	Increased temperature	Heat stroke; sometimes with seizures or head injuries
	Increased sweat rate	Vasovagal reaction; orthostatic hypotension; cardiac
	Profuse sweating	Exertional heat stroke

*See Table 1-2 for normal data

Table 2-6

Mental Status Evaluation[11,12]

AVPU (Alert, Responds to Verbal or Painful stimuli, or Unresponsive) as indicated (Table 1-3).
Glasgow Coma Scale as needed and if time permits (Table 1-7).
Orientation to person, time, and place (Table 1-6).
Retrograde amnesia (loss of memory and events that occurred prior to the injury)—ask the athlete:
- What do you do on a certain play? (The clinician would need to ask about a specific play.)
- Do you know what play was run when the injury occurred?
- Do you know the score of the game?
- Do you know what team you played in the preceding game?
  Post-traumatic amnesia (loss of memory and events that occur after the injury)—
  ask the athlete:
- What do you first recall after the injury?
- Name four objects and have the athlete repeat them back immediately and 5 minutes later.
  Ability to concentrate:
- Name the months of the year backward.
- Count backward from 100, in multiples of 3.
  General impression after the evaluation:
- Facial expression: vacant stare or dazed look.
- Level of consciousness:
  - Alert: aware and responds appropriately and quickly to questions asked.
  - Lethargic: drowsy and falls asleep, but is easily aroused.
  - Stuporous: asleep most of the time and difficult to arouse; inappropriately responds to verbal stimuli.
  - Semicomatose: no response to verbal stimuli, but some reflexive response to pain.
  - Comatose: no response to verbal or painful stimuli; no motor activity.
- Speech patterns.
- Emotional state.

Table 2-7
SAMPLE History

Question	Interpretation
Symptoms	
Ask spectators if there were any tonic or clonic movements (Table 2-2).	Seizure
Did the athlete experience any auras (smells or visions)?	Seizure
Did the athlete experience any palpitations (sensation of skipped beats), chest tightness, or dyspnea?	Cardiogenic
Was there any dizziness or fainting in the weeks prior to the collapse?	Cardiogenic; neurological
Was there any chest pain?	Cardiogenic; pulmonary
Was there an increased breathing rate with numbness in the hands or feet?	Hyperventilation
Were there any feelings of faintness, nausea, light-headedness, or sweating?	Vasovagal reaction; orthostatic hypotension
Are there any injuries associated with the collapse?	Possible hysterical syncope if none (after ruling out all other causes first)
Allergies	
Asthma	Hypoxia
Insect stings	Anaphylactic shock
Exercise	Anaphylactic shock
Certain foods, drugs, or environmental conditions	Anaphylactic shock
Medications	
What current medications are being used?	Several possibilities
Has the athlete recently started any new medications?	Several possibilities
Has the athlete changed the dose of previous medications?	Several possibilities
Is the athlete using any recreational drugs?	Depressants: orthostatic hypotension; Stimulants: cardiac dysrhythmia
Is the athlete using any stimulant drugs to enhance performance?	Cardiac dysrhythmia
Past Medical History	
Is there a history of seizures?	Seizure
Is there a history of cardiac disorders?	Cardiogenic
Is there a family history of sudden death, early heart attack, hyper-cholesterolemia, or congenital heart disease?	Cardiogenic
Has there been a current illness associated with a fever?	Possible myocarditis; cardiogenic syncope
Is there any prior syncope?	Cardiogenic; neurological; hysterical
Is there any recent illness that is associated with vomiting or diarrhea?	Hypotension; metabolic
Has there been any recent head trauma?	Intracerebral vascular accidents
In females, is there the possibility of pregnancy?	Several possibilities
Does the athlete have diabetes?	Hypoglycemia
• Does he or she feel hypoglycemic?	
• Has he or she changed insulin dose or eating or training habits?	
Has there been any recent hemorrhage?	Hypotension
• Recent abdominal injuries?	
• Blood in the urine or stool?	
• Heavy menstruation?	
• Recent injury with significant bleeding?	
Does the athlete have hypertension?	Hypotension secondary to medication
Last Meal Consumed	
When and what was the last meal consumed prior to the sporting event of collapse?	Hypoglycemia
Does the athlete have an eating disorder or abnormal diet?	Hypoglycemia; metabolic
Is the athlete trying to "cut weight?"	Hypoglycemia; metabolic
What is the athlete's hydration status?	Hypovolemia
Events Preceding Injury	
Did the collapse occur during exercise?	Cardiogenic
Did the collapse occur after exercise?	Cardiogenic; heat

Table 2-7, continued

Question	Interpretation
	syncope; post-exercise vasovagal reaction
Did the collapse occur without warning?	Cardiogenic
Did the collapse occur after urination, defecation, coughing, or sneezing?	Vasovagal via valsalva maneuver
Were there any feelings of strong emotions (sight of blood, pain, or fright) prior to the collapse?	Vasovagal
What were the environmental factors prior to the collapse?	Anaphylaxis; asthma
What position was the athlete in just prior to the collapse?	Standing may implicate orthostatic hypotension or vasovagal reaction
Did a blow to the head precede the syncope?	Head injury
Has there been a recent blow to the head in the past few weeks?	Head injury (subdural hematoma)

Table 2-8

Cranial Nerve Evaluation

Cranial Nerve	Functions	Test
I. Olfactory	Smell	Close eyes and identify smells with each nostril.
II. Optic	1. Visual acuity	1. Identify number of fingers held up or read.
	2. Visual fields	2. Approach the athlete's eyes from the side with the athlete looking straight ahead to assess range of visual field.
III. Oculomotor	1. Pupil response	1. Pupil reaction to light.
	2. Medial and superior eye movement	2. Athlete to follow clinician's finger with the eyes only, in medial then superior, and lateral then superior directions.
IV. Trochlear	Moves the eye inferiorly when it is adducted	Athlete to follow clinician's finger using only the eyes, first in a medial, then inferior direction.
V. Trigeminal	1. Facial sensory	1. Assess for light touch sensation over the face.
	2. Motor-mastication	2. Have the athlete clench his or her mouth closed while the examiner palpates for muscle tone over the posterior jaw.
VI. Abducens	Lateral eye movement	Athlete to follow the clinician's finger with the eyes only in a medial and lateral direction.
VII. Facial	1. Facial motor	Have the athlete wrinkle the forehead, smile, wink, and puff cheeks.
	2. Taste (anterior 2/3 of tongue)	
VIII. Vestibulo-cochlear nerves (acoustic)	1. Hearing	1. Clinician rubs fingers together next to athlete's ears and moves fingers outward until the patient can no longer hear them. Compare the hearing distance of both ears.
	2. Balance	2. Romberg's test (Table 3-7).
IX. Glosspharyngeal	1. Swallowing	1. Have the athlete swallow.
	2. Gag reflex	2. Touch back of throat with tongue blade for gag reflex.
	3. Phonation	3. Have the athlete say "ah" while looking for uvula and soft palate midline elevation.
	4. Taste (posterior 1/3 of tongue)	
X. Vagus	1. Swallowing	1. Have the athlete swallow.
	2. Gag reflex	2. Touch back of throat with tongue blade for gag reflex.
XI. Spinal or accessory	Cervical motor	Clinician applies resistance to shoulder shrug and neck rotation.
XII. Hypoglossal	Tongue movement	Clinician attempts to move the athlete's protruding tongue using a tongue blade.

Table 2-9

Motor-Sensory Evaluation[4,6]

Motor Tests
- For dysfunctions of the cerebellum, spinal cord, peripheral nerves, and/or cerebrum/upper motor neurons
- Normal muscle tone: Palpation and passive range of motion to test for rigidity or flaccidness
- Test strength of major muscle groups

Sensation Tests
- For dysfunctions of the spinal cord, peripheral nerves, and/or cerebrum/higher sensory pathways
- Test light touch sensation of extremities and trunk

Reflexes
- For dysfunctions of the spinal cord, peripheral nerves, muscles, and/or cerebrum/higher pathways
- Deep tendon reflexes: biceps, brachioradialis, triceps, quadriceps, and achilles tendons

Coordination Tests
- For dysfunctions of the motor, cerebellar, vestibular, and/or sensory systems
- Romberg's Test: have the athlete stand with the feet together, hands at sides, and eyes open. Then have the athlete close the eyes. The test is positive if the athlete sways back and forth or falls to one side.
- Finger to nose test: with the eyes closed, have the athlete touch his nose with alternating forefingers and with increasing speed. The test is positive if the nose is not consistently touched.
- Heel to knee test: in supine, have the athlete alternatively touch the ground and contralateral knee with the heel. The test is positive if the patella is not consistently touched.

Table 2-10

Cardiovascular Syncope

Cause	History/Precipitating Factors	Prodromal Signs/Symptoms	Postural Association	Rapid Return of Mental Status
Cardiogenic: Types 1. Structural/mechanical 2. Electrical/dysrhythmias	1. Previous syncope 2. Family or personal history of cardiac dysfunctions 3. Stimulant drug use 4. Can occur during or after exercise	Usually none, but if present: 1. Palpitations 2. Fatigue 3. Angina 4. Exertional dyspnea	None	Yes
Orthostatic hypotension: Types 1. Autonomic nervous system (ANS) dysfunctions 2. Medications (antihypertension and depression, pain medications) 3. Heat syncope 4. Hypovolemia	1. History of ANS dysfunctions are present: 2. Currently taking medications for hypertension, depression, or pain 3. Heat syncope due to pooling of blood in lower extremities after exhaustive exercise 4. Hypovolemia due to hemorrhage, gastroenteritis (diarrhea or vomiting), or dehydration (excessive sweating, eating disorders, fasting)	Usually some of the following: 1. Faintness 2. Nausea 3. Diaphoresis (sweating) 4. Pallor 5. Visual dimming 6. Weakness 7. Impaired hearing 8. Hyperventilation	Standing	Yes
Vasovagal reaction: Types 1. Direct vagal nerve stimulation 2. Emotional stimulation 3. Post-exercise 4. Valsalva maneuver followed by a secondary reaction of decreased heart rate and blood pressure	1. Direct vagal nerve stimulation due to a blow to the stomach (solar plexus) or eye 2. Emotional stimulation due to fright, pain, sight of blood 3. Post-exercise strong ventricular contractions that stimulate the afferent input to the vasovagal reaction 4. Valsalva maneuver due to coughing, sneezing, defecation, or urination	Usually same as for orthostatic hypotension	Standing	Yes

Table 2-10, continued

Cause	History/ Precipitating Factors	Prodromal Signs/Symptoms	Postural Association	Rapid Return of Mental Status
Weightlifter's syncope: Any combination of 1. Orthostatic hypotension 2. Valsalva maneuver 3. Hyperventilation	Intense weightlifting, usually with the lower extremities	Usually same as for orthostatic hypotension	Standing	Yes

Table 2-11
Noncardiovascular Syncope

Cause	History/ Precipitating Factors	Prodromal Signs/Symptoms	Postural Association	Rapid Return of Mental Status
Neurogenic: Types 1. Concussion 2. Intracranial hemorrhage 3. Cerebral vascular disruption 4. Neoplasm	1. Blow to the head by an object or the ground 2. Vascular anomaly 3. Cancer	Usually none See Chapter 3	None	No
Metabolic: Types 1. Hyperventilation	Hypocapnia (abnormally low level of carbon dioxide in the blood): 1. Extreme exercise 2. Emotional stress	1. Chest pain 2. Numbness of hands, feet, and lips	None	Yes
2. Hypoglycemia (abnormally low levels of glucose in the blood)	1. Diabetes: • Too much insulin intake • Too much exercise • Not enough glucose intake 2. Exhaustive exercise > 60 minutes without glucose supplementation	Early phase: 1. Sweating 2. Tremor 3. Tachycardia 4. Anxiety 5. Hunger Late phase:	None	Yes, if caught in early phase and glucose is given. Otherwise, no.

Table 2-11, continued

Cause	History/Precipitating Factors	Prodromal Signs/Symptoms	Postural Association	Rapid Return of Mental Status
	3. Eating disorder or cutting weight	1. Dizzy 2. Headache 3. Confusion 4. Convulsions 5. Coma		
3. Hypoxia (reduction of an adequate oxygen supply to the tissues in the presence of normal blood flow)	1. Airway obstruction: • Objects • Throat swelling 2. Asthma: • See Chapter 11 3. Pulmonary embolism: • Recent surgery or immobilization 4. Third-stage anemia: • History of anemia	1. Confusion 2. Agitation 3. Impaired judgment 4. Poor motor coordination	None	Variable
4. Hyponatremia (abnormally low level of sodium in the urine, which is rare in athletes)	1. Water intoxication: • Drinking excessive hypotonic solutions during intensive exercise 2. Poor sodium intake: • Eating disorder	1. Altered mental status 2. Confusion 3. Seizures 4. Coma	None	No
5. Hypokalemia (abnormally low level of potassium in the blood, which is rare in athletes)	1. Many underlying disorders 2. In athletes: • Gastroenteritis with diarrhea or vomiting • Low dietary intake due to eating disorder/fasting	1. Muscle weakness: • Skeletal • Respiratory • Smooth muscle in digestive system • Myocardium 2. Palpitations 3. Diminished deep tendon reflexes	None	No
6. Hypocalcemia (abnormally low level of calcium in the blood, which is rare in athletes)	1. Many underlying disorders 2. In athletes: • Low vitamin D intake due to eating disorder/fasting	1. Palpitations	None	No
Anaphylactic reaction:	1. Known anaphylactic reaction: insect stings, certain foods, exercise (see Chapter 11)	1. Respiratory distress 2. Nausea 3. Vomiting 4. Dizziness 5. Sweating 6. Fever 7. Rhinitis 8. Hypotension		

Table 2-11, Continued

Cause	History/ Precipitating Factors	Prodromal Signs/Symptoms	Postural Association	Rapid Return of Mental Status
Heat stroke: 1. Hypovolemia 2. TLOC to allow body temperature to decrease 3. See Chapter 10	1. Exercising in high ambient temperatures 2. Poor hydration	1. Profuse or lack of sweating 2. Headache 3. Confusion 4. Disorientation 5. Drowsiness	None	Usually not
Psychotic disorders: (faked syncope due to hysterical reaction)	1. Multiple syncope attacks without any associated injuries from the falls	1. Bizarre symptoms	None	Variable

References

1. Shen WK. The fainting athlete: when is it a heart problem? Your patient and fitness. *Phys Sportsmed.* 1997;26(2):26j-26v.
2. Wang D, Sakaguchi S, Babcock M. Exercise-induced vasovagal syncope. *Phys Sportsmed.* 1997;25(5):64-74.
3. Cantwell JD, Varughese A, Pettus CW. Cardiovascular syncope. *Phys Sportsmed.* 1992;20(1):81-92.
4. Hargarten K. Syncope in athletes: finding the cause in active people. *Phys Sportsmed.* 1992;20(5):123-141.
5. Preblick-Salib C, Jagoda A. Spells: differential diagnosis and management strategies. *Emer Med Clin N Amer.* 1997;15:637-648.
6. Rund, DA. Syncope. *Phys Sportsmed.* 1990;18(7):141-142.
7. Williams CC, Bernhardt DT. Syncope in athletes. *Sports Med.* 1995;19: 223-234.
8. Adams RD, Martin JB. Faintness, syncope, and seizures. In: Braunwald E, Isselbacher KJ, Petersdorf RG, Wilson JD, Martin JB, Fauci AS, eds. *Harrison's Principles of Internal Medicine. 11th ed.* New York, NY: McGraw-Hill Book Co; 1988:64-70.
9. Booher J, Thibodeau G. *Athletic Injury Assessment. 3rd ed.* St. Louis, Mo: Mosby; 1994:88-115, 266-289, 316-353.
10. Torg JS, Ramsey-Emrhein JA. Cervical spine and brachial plexus injuries. *Phys Sportsmed.* 1997;25(7):61-88.
11. American Academy of Neurology. Practice parameter: the management of concussion in sports (summary statement). *Neurology.* 1997;48:581-585.
12. Price MB, DeVroom HL. A quick and easy guide to neurological assessment. *J Neurosurg Nurs.* 1985;17:313-320.
13. Bates B, Bickley LS, Hoekelman RA. *A Guide to Physical Examination and History Taking. 6th ed.* Philadelphia, Pa: JB Lippincott Co; 1991:90-91, 491-554.

Bibliography

Armstrong LE, et al. Voluntary dehydration and electrolyte losses during prolonged exercise in the heat. *Aviation, Space, Environ Med.* 1985;Aug:765-770.

Bell JA, Doege TC. Athletes' use and abuse of drugs. *Phys Sportsmed.* 1987;15(3):99-108.

Braunwald E. Cyanosis, hypoxia, and polycythemia. In: Braunwald E, Isselbacher KJ, Petersdorf RG, Wilson JD, Martin JB, Fauci AS, eds. *Harrison's Principles of Internal Medicine. 11th ed.* New York, NY: McGraw-Hill Book Co; 1988:145-153.

Bunn HF. Anemia. In: Braunwald E, Isselbacher KJ, Petersdorf RG, Wilson JD, Martin JB, Fauci AS, eds. *Harrison's Principles of Internal Medicine. 11th ed.* New York, NY: McGraw-Hill Book Co; 1988:262-266.

Ciccone CD. *Pharmacology in Rehabilitation.* Philadelphia, Pa: FA Davis Co; 1990:81-89.

Colucciello SA, Plotka M. Abdominal trauma: occult injury may be life threatening. *Phys Sportsmed.* 1993;21(6):33-43.

Costill DL, Cote R, Fink W. Muscle water and electrolytes following varied levels of dehydration in man. *J Appl Phys.* 1976;40:6-11.

Felig P, Cherif A, Minagawa A, Wahren J. Hypoglycemia during prolonged exercise in normal men. *N Engl J Med.* 1982;306:895-900.

Foster DW, Rubenstein AH. Hypoglycemia, insulinoma, and other hormone-secreting tumors of the pancreas. In: Braunwald E, Isselbacher KJ, Petersdorf RG, Wilson JD, Martin JB, Fauci AS, eds. *Harrison's Principles of Internal Medicine. 11th ed.* New York, NY: McGraw-Hill Book Co; 1988:1800-1807.

Gennarelli TA. Cerebral concussion and diffuse brain injuries. In: Torg JS, ed. *Athletic Injuries to the Head, Neck, and Face. 2nd ed.* St. Louis, Mo: Mosby-Year Book; 1991:270-282.

Hubbard RW, Armstrong LE. Hyperthermia: new thoughts on an old problem. *Phys Sportsmed.* 1989;17(6):97-113.

Kizer KW. Treating insect stings. *Phys Sportsmed.* 1991;19(8):33-36.

Leizman DJ, Mosley GM, Byrd JC. Case report: frontal astrcytoma—a cause of exertional syncope? *Phys Sportsmed.* 1992;20(3):181-186..

Levinsky NG. Acidosis and alkalosis. In: Braunwald E, Isselbacher KJ, Petersdorf RG, Wilson JD, Martin JB, Fauci AS, eds. *Harrison's Principles of Internal Medicine. 11th ed.* New York, NY: McGraw-Hill Book Co; 1988:208-214.

Levinsky NG. Fluids and electrolytes. In: Braunwald E, Isselbacher KJ, Petersdorf RG, Wilson JD, Martin JB, Fauci AS, eds. *Harrison's Principles of Internal Medicine. 11th ed.* New York, NY: McGraw-Hill Book Co; 1988:198-208.

Mahler DA. Exercise-induced asthma. *Med Sci Sport Exer.* 1993;25:554-561.

Martin GJ, Adams SL, Martin HG. Prospective evaluation of syncope. *Ann Emer Med.* 1984;13:499-504.

Montain SJ, Maughan RJ, Sawka MN. Fluid replacement strategies for exercise in hot weather. *Athletic Therapy Today.* 1996;1(4):24-27.

Moser KM. Pulmonary thromboembolism. In: Braunwald E, Isselbacher KJ, Petersdorf RG, Wilson JD, Martin JB, Fauci AS, eds. *Harrison's Principles of Internal Medicine. 11th ed.* New York, NY: McGraw-Hill Book Co; 1988:1105-1111.

Nelson PB, Robinson AG, Kapoor W, Rinaldo J. Case report: hyponatremia in a marathoner. *Phys Sportsmed.* 1988;16(10):78-87.

Noakes TD, Norman RJ, Buck RH, Godlonton J, Stevenson K, Pitway D. The incidence of hyponatremia during prolonged ultraendurance exercise. *Med Sci Sport Exer.* 1990;22:165-170.

Puffer JC, Green GA. Drugs and doping in athletes. In: Mellion MB, Walsh WM, Shelton GL, eds. *The Team Physician's Handbook.* Philadelphia, Pa: Hanley & Belfus, Inc; 1990:111-127.

Rund DA. Airway obstruction: recognition and immediate management. *Phys Sportsmed.* 1989;17(10):173-174.

Rund DA. Asthma. *Phys Sportsmed.* 1990;18(1):143-146.

Sandor RP. Heat illness: on-site diagnosis and cooling. *Phys Sportsmed.* 1997;25(6):35-40.

Schwenk TS. Psychoactive drugs and athletic performance. *Phys Sportsmed.* 1997;25(1):32-46.

Selby GB. When does an athlete need iron? *Phys Sportsmed.* 1991;19(4):96-102.

Shapiro Y, Seidman DS. Field and clinical observations of exertional heat stroke patients. *Med Sci Sports Exer.* 1990;22:6-14.

Siven JI, Varrato J. Physical activity and epilepsy. *Phys Sportsmed.* 1999;27(3):63-70.

Taunton JE, McCargar L. Managing activity in patients who have diabetes. *Phys Sportsmed.* 1995;23(3):41-52.

Taylor L. Preventing disordered eating in athletics. *Athletic Therapy Today.* 1997;2(2):33-36.

Terrell TT, Hough DO, Alexander R. Identifying exercise allergies. *Phys Sportsmed.* 1996;24(11):76-89.

Thein LA. Environmental conditions affecting the athlete. *JOSPT.* 1995;21:158-171.

Wise SL, Stafford CT. Anaphylaxis from exercise. *Emer Med.* 1991;June(15):141-144.

CHAPTER 3

Head Injuries

In all sports, there is a risk of injury that can harm the brain. However, some sports such as football, horseback riding, and bicycling have higher risks. Although most brain injuries are minor in nature, some can be serious and life threatening.[1] Brain injuries (also called head injuries) are the leading cause of death in athletes.[2] Brain injuries can be divided into concussions and intracranial hemorrhaging. A concussion is a traumatically induced alteration in mental status with or without a loss of consciousness.[3] When a loss of consciousness occurs, it is due to an alteration in the normal function of the reticular activating system. The reticular activating system is the neurophysiological system that originates at the brainstem and connects to the cerebrum; it is responsible for maintaining consciousness. Mild and moderate concussions involve damage to the neurons inside the brain. In severe concussions, edema and swelling in the brain can also occur. The signs and symptoms of a concussion can last weeks or months. Postconcussion syndrome is the persistence of signs and symptoms after a concussion including headaches, fatigue, irritability, amnesia, and lack of concentration. Intracranial hemorrhaging includes bleeding inside the brain, or bleeding that occurs between the meninges. The meninges are the protective covering of the brain. From superficial to deep, they include the dura mater, arachnoid membrane, and the pia mater.

Second-impact syndrome can also be considered a type of head injury. Second-impact syndrome can develop when a second head injury occurs before the signs and symptoms of the first head injury have completely resolved. In second-impact syndrome, the autoregulation of profusion to the brain is disrupted, which causes an increase in blood flow to the brain. This leads to rapid brain swelling, increased intracranial pressure, and herniation of brain matter through the large hole at the base of the skull (foramen magna). The neurological status of the athlete quickly deteriorates over several minutes, which can lead to death.[4,5]

There is much debate and confusion on how to classify the severity of a concussion. Several classifications have been developed. Table 3-1 describes the most commonly used concussion classifications. Also, there are no universally accepted protocols for assessing athletes with head injuries, although some investigators are currently trying to develop some.[6] For safety purposes, the most conservative parameters were used in developing the algorithm for this chapter. The algorithm is designed to help the clinician differentiate between mild and more serious problems. A mild first-occurrence concussion that is self-limiting can usually be treated on the sidelines. However, the suspicion of more serious problems, such as a repeated concussion, a mild concussion with persistent signs and symptoms, a more severe concussion, or an intracranial hemorrhage, need to be referred for a medical evaluation.

There are four basic mechanisms that can cause a head injury.[7,8] First, an injury can occur at the site of impact (coup injury) when a resting, moveable head receives a blow. Second, an injury can occur at the opposite side of impact (contracoup), when a head in motion contacts an immovable object (ie, head hitting the ground). Third, in the event of a skull fracture, a brain injury can occur at the site of the fracture. Fourth, diffuse brain injuries can occur with acceleration and deceleration movements, primarily in a rotational manor, which can cause damaging tension forces on the axons in the brain.

The most common sites of brain injury are the midbrain and the frontal and temporal lobes.[2,8] The frontal and temporal lobes have the deepest sulci and gyri. Additionally, the floor of the skull can be irregular under these areas. Therefore, the least amount of free movement between the brain and skull is at these sites. This is a reason why brain injuries commonly occur in the frontal and temporal lobes. With the brain swelling and/or hemorrhaging that can occur with a brain injury, the brain stem (medulla, pons, and midbrain), which contain the cranial nerve cell bodies, can be forced through and against the foramen magna. Also, during a brain injury there can be a shearing force between the mobile cerebral cortex and the relatively immobile brain stem, which can injure the reticular activating system. Therefore, signs and symptoms of damage to the frontal lobe (impairment and weakness of voluntary movement, cognitive changes, sensory changes), temporal lobe (slurred speech, nausea, depressed visual and auditory memory), reticular activating system, (decreased level of consciousness), and brain stem (decreased level of consciousness, autonomic changes, cranial nerve dysfunctions) are primarily evaluated when assessing for a head injury. However, remember that a local injury can occur at the specific site of an impact to the head; in this situation, the signs and symptoms would be specific to the site of brain injury.

When evaluating an athlete with a possible head injury, the clinician must keep several things in mind. First, always assume the presence of a head injury when a mechanism of injury involves a blow to the head, an acceleration/deceleration injury, or when a laceration to the head is present.[9,10] Second, when evaluating for a head injury, first assume the possibility of a cervical spine injury. The cervical spine should be immobilized until a cervical spine injury is ruled out. A cervical spine injury should be assumed when an athlete presents with a decreased level of consciousness.[2,10] Third, 90% of concussions are mild and usually escape a medical evaluation.[2] Therefore, it is important to carefully evaluate for a head injury whenever one is suspected. In these individuals, the signs and symptoms of a head injury may be so slight that they can only be detected by performing a detailed and thorough evaluation. The mental status exam is the most important aspect of a head injury evaluation.[2] It is important to realize that lack of an initial loss of consciousness does not always correlate with the seriousness of a head injury. An athlete can be unconscious for a few seconds, which could be classified as a benign first- or second-degree concussion. Another athlete could never loose consciousness while suffering from an subdural hematoma, which is a life-threatening emergency.[9] Fifth, an athlete who has a head injury should never be allowed to return to practice or play until all signs and symptoms are completely resolved. Even if the signs and symptoms completely resolve, serial re-evaluations must be performed in the following weeks. This is because an intracranial hematoma can develop over a period of minutes or even weeks; a patient with a head injury should be closely evaluated for 24 hours after the injury, and even up to several weeks post injury. Lastly, a physician should evaluate an injured athlete if he or she has loss of consciousness, deteriorating neurological status, and/or suspicion of an intracranial hemorrhage, or has signs and symptoms of a first-degree concussion longer then 20 to 30 minutes.

EVALUATION OF A HEAD INJURY

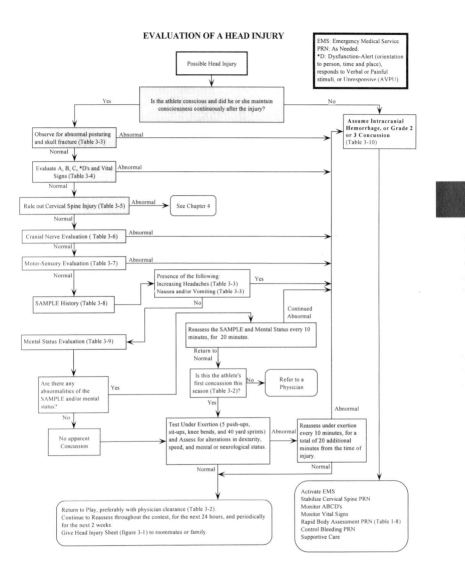

EMS: Emergency Medical Service.
PRN: As Needed.
*D: Dysfunction-Alert (orientation to person, time and place), responds to Verbal or Painful stimuli, or Unresponsive (AVPU)

Possible Head Injury

Is the athlete conscious and did he or she maintain consciousness continuously after the injury?

Yes — Observe for abnormal posturing and skull fracture (Table 3-3)

No — **Assume Intracranial Hemorrhage, or Grade 2 or 3 Concussion** (Table 3-10)

Abnormal →

Normal — Evaluate A, B, C, *D's and Vital Signs (Table 3-4)
Abnormal →
Normal — Rule out Cervical Spine Injury (Table 3-5)
Abnormal → See Chapter 4
Normal — Cranial Nerve Evaluation (Table 3-6)
Abnormal →
Normal — Motor-Sensory Evaluation (Table 3-7)
Abnormal →
Normal — SAMPLE History (Table 3-8)

Presence of the following:
Increasing Headaches (Table 3-3)
Nausea and/or Vomiting (Table 3-3)
Yes →
No

Continued Abnormal

Reassess the SAMPLE and Mental Status every 10 minutes, for 20 minutes.

Return to Normal

Mental Status Evaluation (Table 3-9)

Is this the athlete's first concussion this season (Table 3-2)?
No → Refer to a Physician
Yes

Are there any abnormalities of the SAMPLE and/or mental status?
Yes →
No

No apparent Concussion

Test Under Exertion (5 push-ups, sit-ups, knee bends, and 40 yard sprints) and Assess for alterations in dexterity, speed, and mental or neurological status.
Abnormal →
Reassess under exertion every 10 minutes, for a total of 20 additional minutes from the time of injury.
Abnormal →

Normal

Normal

Return to Play, preferably with physician clearance (Table 3-2).
Continue to Reassess throughout the contest, for the next 24 hours, and periodically for the next 2 weeks.
Give Head Injury Sheet (figure 3-1) to roommates or family.

Activate EMS
Stabilize Cervical Spine PRN
Monitor ABCD's
Monitor Vital Signs
Rapid Body Assessment PRN (Table 1-8)
Control Bleeding PRN
Supportive Care

Table 3-1

Classification of Concussion Severity

Grade	Cantu Guidelines[3]	Colorado Guidelines[4]	American Academy of Neurology[11]
1. Mild	No loss of consciousness Post-traumatic amnesia less than 30 minutes	No loss of consciousness Confusion without amnesia	No loss of consciousness Symptoms or mental status abnormalities less than 15 minutes
2. Moderate	Loss of consciousness less than 5 minutes Post-traumatic amnesia greater than 30 minutes	No loss of consciousness Confusion with amnesia	No loss of consciousness Transient confusion Symptoms of mental status abnormalities more than 15 minutes
3. Severe	Loss of consciousness greater than 5 minutes Post-traumatic amnesia greater than 24 hours	Loss of consciousness	Loss of consciousness

Table 3-2

Cantu Guidelines for Return to Play After Concussion

Grade	First Concussion	Second Concussion	Third Concussion
1. Mild	May return to play if asymptomatic*	Return to play in 2 weeks if asymptomatic for 1 week	Terminate season; may return to play next season if asymptomatic
2. Moderate	Return to play after asymptomatic for 1 week	Minimum of 1 month; may then return to play if asymptomatic for 1 week; consider terminating season	Terminate season; may return to play next season if asymptomatic
3. Severe	Minimum of 1 month no play; may then return to play if asymptomatic for 1 week	Terminate season; may return to play next season if asymptomatic	N/A

*No headache, dizziness, or impaired orientation, concentration, or memory during rest or exertion.

From Cantu RC. Cantu guidelines for return to play after a concussion. *Phys Sportsmed.* 1986;14(10). Reprinted with permission from McGraw-Hill Co.

Table 3-3

Some Signs and Symptoms of a Head Injury Requiring Immediate Medical Referral

Intracranial Hemorrhage[12]

- Increasing headache
- Nausea or vomiting
- Pupil irregularity
- Localizing neurological deficits
- Confusion
- Progressive impairment of consciousness
- Sudden unconsciousness
- Rising blood pressure
- Falling pulse rate
- Abnormal breathing rhythm

Abnormal Posturing

- Decerebrate: extension of all four extremities (midbrain or brainstem injury)
- Decorticate: extension of lower extremities; adduction, flexion of the elbow, wrist, and fingers (diencephalon injury)

Possible Skull Fracture

- Abnormalities, crepitation, and/or step-off with palpation
- Otorrhea: discharge from the ears (blood or cerebrospinal fluid)
- Rhinorrhea: discharge from the nose (blood or cerebrospinal fluid)
- Raccoon sign: discoloration of the eyelids and periorbital region (orbital or basilar skull fracture)
- Battle's sign: discoloration over the mastoid process (temporal or basilar skull fracture)

Make an immediate medical referral whenever in doubt regarding the seriousness of the injury.

Table 3-4

Vital Signs—Possible Abnormal Findings in the Presence of a Head Injury*

Vital Sign	Abnormality
Pulse	Slow and strong
Breathing—rhythms	Central neurogenic hyperventilation: rapid deep pattern
	Cheyne-Strokes pattern: increasing and decreasing rate and depth/volume
	Biot's respiration: irregular pattern of apnea and hyper-ventilation
Blood pressure	Increasing systolic with same or decreasing diastolic
Pupil reaction	Dilated and fixed
	Anisocoria: unequal pupil reactions
	Doll's eye response: eyes move with head during rotation (not to be tested if suspected cervical spine injury)
	Presence of nystagmus (involuntary rapid movement of the eyeballs)

*See Table 1-2 for normal data.

Table 3-5

Some Signs and Symptoms of a Significant Cervical Spine Injury[1,13]

- Involuntary loss of bowel and/or bladder control
- Cervical pain without movement
- Pain with palpation over the posterior or anterior cervical spine
- Rigid muscle spasms of the anterior and/or posterior neck muscles
- Deformity detected by palpation or the presence of a wryneck (abnormal neck position usually including flexion, rotation, and side bending)
- Decreased cervical spine mobility with pain
- Persistent burning, weakness, tingling, or numbness in any extremity

Table 3-6

Cranial Nerve Evaluation

Cranial Nerve	Functions	Test
I. Olfactory	Smell	Close eyes and identify smells with each nostril.
II. Optic	1. Visual acuity	1. Identify number of fingers held up or read.
	2. Visual fields	2. Approach the athlete's eyes from the side with the athlete looking straight ahead to assess range of visual field.
III. Oculomotor	1. Pupil response	1. Pupil reaction to light.
	2. Medial and superior eye movement	2. Athlete to follow clinician's finger with the eyes only in medial then superior, and lateral then superior directions.
IV. Trochlear	Moves the eye inferiorly when it is adducted	Athlete to follow clinician's finger using only the eyes first in a medial, then inferior direction.
V. Trigeminal	1. Facial sensory	1. Assess for light touch sensation over the face.
	2. Motor-mastication	2. Have the athlete clench his or her mouth closed while the examiner palpates for muscle tone over the posterior jaw.
VI. Abducens	Lateral eye movement	Athlete to follow the clinician's finger with the eyes only in a medial and lateral direction.
VII. Facial	1. Facial motor	Have the athlete wrinkle the forehead, smile, wink, and puff cheeks.
	2. Taste (anterior 2/3 of tongue)	
VIII. Vestibulo-cochlear nerves (acoustic)	1. Hearing	1. Clinician rubs fingers together next to athlete's ears and moves fingers outward until the patient can no longer hear them. Compare the hearing distance of both ears.
	2. Balance	2. Romberg's test.
IX. Glosspharyngeal	1. Swallowing	1. Have the athlete swallow.
	2. Gag reflex	2. Touch back of throat with tongue blade for gag reflex.
	3. Phonation	3. Have the athlete say "ah" while looking for uvula and soft palate midline elevation.
	4. Taste (posterior 1/3 of tongue)	
X. Vagus	1. Swallowing	1. Have the athlete swallow.
	2. Gag reflex	2. Touch back of throat with tongue blade for gag reflex.
XI. Spinal or accessory	Cervical motor	Clinician applies resistance to shoulder shrug and neck rotation.
XII. Hypoglossal	Tongue movement	Clinician attempts to move the athlete's protruding tongue using a tongue blade.

Table 3-7
Motor-Sensory Evaluation*

Motor Tests (for dysfunctions of the cerebellum, spinal cord, peripheral nerves, and/or cerebrum/upper motor neurons):
- Normal muscle tone: palpation and passive range of motion to test for rigidity or flaccidness.
- Test strength of major muscle groups.

Sensation Tests (for dysfunctions of the spinal cord, peripheral nerves, and/or cerebrum/higher sensory pathways):
- Test light touch sensation of extremities and trunk.

Reflex Tests (for dysfunctions of the spinal cord, peripheral nerves, muscles, and/or cerebrum/higher pathways):
- Deep tendon reflexes: biceps, brachioradialis, triceps, quadriceps, and Achilles tendons.

Coordination Tests (for dysfunctions of the motor, cerebellar, vestibular, and/or sensory systems):
- Romberg's test: have the athlete stand with the feet together, hands at sides, and eyes open. Then have the athlete close the eyes. The test is positive if the patient sways back and forth or falls to one side.
- Finger to nose test: with the eyes closed, have the athlete touch his or her nose with alternating forefingers and with increasing speed. The test is positive if the nose is not consistently touched.
- Heel to knee test: in supine, have the athlete alternatively touch the ground and contralateral knee with the heel. The test is positive if the patella is not consistently touched.

*Primarily assessed in this chapter for a lesion to the motor or sensory systems of the brain.[1,14]

Table 3-8
SAMPLE History

Question	Interpretation
Symptoms	
Do you have any of the following: headache, dizziness, nausea, vomiting, ringing in the ears, sensitivity to light, difficulty concentrating, double or blurred vision?	All are signs and symptoms of a significant head injury.
Allergies	
Do you have any known allergies?	Knowledge of allergies may be helpful to a physician or paramedic.
Medications	
Are you currently taking any nonsteroidal anti-inflammatory medications?	These medications could increase intracranial hemorrhaging.
Are you taking any antidepressant or hypertensive medications?	These medications could possibly cause some of the aforementioned signs and symptoms.
Past Medical History	
Have you ever suffered a concussion or other head injury; if so, when did it occur?	People with previous head injuries are at increased risk of developing another head injury.
If the answer was yes, have all of the signs and symptoms from the previous head injury completely resolved?	Possible risk of developing second impact syndrome if the signs and symptoms have not resolved from the first head injury.
Last Meal Consumed	
When was the last time that you ate or drank?	This information may be helpful to a physician or paramedic. Also, this is a possible test for retrograde amnesia (loss of memory and events that occurred prior to the injury).
Events Preceding the Injury	
Was there a blow to the head or a fall to the	This is a possible test for retrograde amnesia.

Table 3-9
Mental Status Evaluation[11,15]

AVPU (alert, responds to verbal or painful stimuli, or unresponsive) as indicated (Table 1-3).
Glasgow Coma Scale as needed and if time permits (Table 1-7).
Orientation to person, time, and place (Table 1-6).
Retrograde amnesia (loss of memory and events that occurred prior to the injury)—ask the athlete:
• What do you do on a certain play? (The clinician would need to ask about a specific play.)
• Do you know what play was run when the injury occurred?
• Do you know the score of the game?
• Do you know what team you played in the preceding game?
Post-traumatic amnesia (loss of memory and events that occur after the injury)—ask the athlete:
• What do you first recall after the injury?
• Name four objects and have the athlete repeat them back immediately and 5 minutes later.
Ability to concentrate:
• Name the months of the year backward.
• Count backward from 100 in multiples of 3.
General impression after the evaluation:
• Facial expression: vacant stare or dazed look.
• Level of consciousness:
  • Alert: aware and responds appropriately and quickly to questions asked.
  • Lethargic: drowsy and falls asleep, but is easily aroused.
  • Stuporous: asleep most of the time and difficult to arouse; inappropriately responds to verbal stimuli.
  • Semicomatose: no response to verbal stimuli but some reflexive response to pain.
  • Comatose: no response to verbal or painful stimuli; no motor activity.
• Speech patterns.
• Emotional state.
• Appropriate verbal and nonverbal responses to the above questions.

Table 3-10

Intracranial Conditions

Condition	Mechanism and General Information	Possible Signs/Symptoms
Concussion	1. Disruption of neurons and capillaries in the brainstem and/or reticular activating system 2. Some symptoms develop rapidly such as headache, dizziness, confusion, and nausea 3. Other symptoms (listed to the right) may develop over days or weeks	1. See Table 3-1 2. Hallmark signs are confusion and amnesia 3. Other signs and symptoms include possible loss of consciousness, dizziness, headache, disorientation, slurred speech, poor motor coordination, sensory changes, inability to maintain a stream of thought, photophobia (unusual sensitivity to light), emotionally labile

Second impact syndrome	1. Occurs when an athlete receives a second head injury before the signs and symptoms of the first head injury have resolved
	2. A dysfunction of the cerebral blood supply autoregulation that causes vascular engorgement and secondary intracranial hypertension
	3. The second blow may be mild or even occur to the trunk, which may cause a slight snapping of the neck and head
		1. The athlete initially looks stunned
		2. Usually no initial loss of consciousness
		3. Neurological deterioration occurs in the next 2 to 5 minutes:
		  • Collapse
		  • Semicomatose
		  • Dilating pupils
		  • Respiratory failure
		  • Possible death

Epidural hematoma	1. Hematoma forms between the skull and the outer brain covering (dura mater)
	2. Associated with a high-force injury and usually with a fracture of the temporal bone
	3. High level of fatality
	4. Needs surgery in 1 to 2 hours post-injury for a favorable outcome
	5. Usually rapidly developing but can develop over a 24-hour period
		1. Usually an initial loss of consciousness
		2. May be followed by a lucent period with a return of consciousness for 15 to 30 minutes
		3. Then, a rapid deterioration of level of consciousness with an increasing headache
		4. One-third of cases have the following hallmark signs:
		  • Ipsilateral dilated pupil
		  • Contralateral muscle weakness
		  • Decerebrate posturing

Subdural hematoma	1. Hematoma between brain surface and the dura mater
	2. Requires less force than an epidural hematoma and is three times more prevalent
	3. Can be acute or chronic
		1. In an acute subdural hematoma, the athlete has an initial loss of consciousness that is not regained
		2. Chronic subdural hematoma:
		  • Develops over days or weeks
		  • Increasing headaches
		  • Slight changes in mental status, motor skills, sensation changes

Subarachnoid hematoma	1. Hematoma on superficial surface of brain ("brain bruise") 2. Can occur due to rupture of brain vessels, aneurysm, or arteriovenous malformation	1. Neurological deficits depend on the area of involvement 2. A severe headache is usually present 3. A lucent period and seizures are possible 4. There is rapid neurological deterioration

Table 3-10, continued

Condition	Mechanism and General Information	Possible Signs/Symptoms
Intracerebral hematoma	1. Hematoma develops deep within brain 2. Same rupture possibilities mentioned for subarachnoid hematoma 3. Death usually occurs prior to arrival to hospital	1. Usually an initial loss of consciousness 2. Usually no lucid period 3. Rapid neurological deterioration
Post-concussion syndrome	Persistent signs and symptoms after a concussion	1. Headache 2. Fatigue 3. Irritability 4. Amnesia 5. Lack of concentration

HEAD INJURY INSTRUCTION SHEET

Date:_____

_____ has suffered a head injury. Although the athlete is currently alert, conscious, and shows no signs or symptoms of a serious brain injury, a potentially catastrophic result can still occur, leading to permanent neurological deficit or even death. Occasionally, following even the mildest head injuries, blood can slowly accumulate, causing compression of the brain hours or even days after the initial injury. Thus, the following guidelines should be followed in conjunction with the advice of the physician, sports physical therapist, or athletic trainer.

1. The injured athlete should not be left alone for the first 24 hours after the injury.
2. The injured athlete should not be allowed to drive for the first 24 hours after the injury.
3. The injured athlete should not consume alcohol for the first 24 hours after the injury.
4. The injured athlete should not take analgesic medications for his or her symptoms (eg, aspirin, ibuprofen, etc).
5. The following signs mandate immediate emergency room evaluation:
   - Blood or watery fluid coming from the ears or nose
   - Unequal or dilated pupils
   - Weakness or clumsiness in arms or legs
   - Slurred or garbled speech
   - Asymmetry of the face
   - Increased swelling along the scalp
   - Hard to arouse, irritable, or stuporous (reduced sensibility)
6. The following symptoms (complaints) mandate immediate emergency room evaluation:
   - Change in mental status (inability to concentrate or understand directions, alteration in alertness or consciousness)
   - Doubled or blurred vision
   - Severe headache
   - Increased incoordination (clumsiness) or weakness
   - Vomiting
   - Loss of memory
   - Difficulty with speech

Please realize the above are only guidelines to assist you. If a sign or symptom develops that is new and is not mentioned above, err on the side of safety and have the athlete evaluated by a physician immediately.

Important Phone Numbers:
Emergency Medical Service: 911 or _____
Team Physician: _____
Sports Physical Therapist or Athletic Trainer: _____

Adapted from Annable B. Concussions. Sports Med Update. *1997;12:11-13. Reprinted with permission from HealthSouth Corp.*

References

1. Fink ME. Head trauma. In: Scuderi G, McCann P, Bruno P, eds. *Sports Medicine: Principles of Primary Care.* St. Louis, Mo: Mosby; 1996:74-85.
2. Cantu RC. Guidelines for return to contact sports after a cerebral concussion. *Phys Sportsmed.* 1986;14(10):75-83.
3. Annable B. Concussions. *Sports Medicine Update.* 1997;12:11-13.
4. Cantu RC. Second-impact syndrome. *Clin Sports Med.* 1998;17:37-44.
5. Kelly JP, Rosenberg JH. Diagnosis and management of concussion in sports. *Neurology.* 1997;48:575-580.
6. McCrea M, Kelly JP, Kluge J, Ackley B, Randolph C. Standardized assessment of concussion in football players. *Neurology.* 1997;48:586-588.
7. Bruno LA. Focal intracranial hematoma. In: Torg JS, ed. *Athletic Injuries to the Head, Neck, and Face. 2nd ed.* St. Louis, Mo: Mosby-Year Book; 1991:305-322.
8. Gallaspy JB, May JD. *Signs and Symptoms of Athletic Injuries.* St. Louis, Mo: Mosby; 1996:23-39.
9. Torg JS, Ramsey-Emrhein JA. Cervical spine and brachial plexus injuries. *Phys Sportsmed.* 1997;25(7):61-88.
10. Vegso JJ, Torg JS. Field evaluation and management of intracranial injuries. In: Torg JS, ed. *Athletic Injuries to the Head, Neck, and Face. 2nd ed.* St. Louis, Mo: Mosby-Year Book; 1991:225-231.
11. Carter RL, Day AL. Head and neck injuries. In: Mellion M, Walsh W, Shelton G, ed. *The Team Physician's Handbook.* Philadelphia, Pa: Hanley & Belfus; 1990:279-288.
12. Colorado Medical Society. *Guidelines for the Management of Concussion in Sports.*
13. Fagan KM. Head and neck injuries. In: Andrews JR, Clancy WG, Whiteside JA, eds. *On-Field Evaluation and Treatment of Common Athletic Injuries.* St. Louis, Mo: Mosby; 1997:1-15.
14. Athletic Training Emergency Care. *Course Notebook.* Wichita, KS, April 1997 (c/o DCH Outpatient Services, 809 University Boulevard East, Tuscaloosa, AL 35401).
15. Cantu RC. Athletic head injuries. *Clin Sports Med.* 1997;16:531-542.

Bibliography

American Academy of Neurology. Practice parameter: the management of concussion in sports (summary statement). *Neurology.* 1997;48:581-585.

Arnheim D. *Modern Principles of Athletic Training.* St. Louis, Mo: Times Mirror/Mosby College Publishing; 1989:711-718.

Barker S. Screening for nervous system disease. In: Boissonnault WG, ed. *Examination in Physical Therapy Practice. 2nd ed.* New York, NY: Churchill Livingstone; 1995:191-222.

Bates B, Bickley LS, Hoekelman RA. *A Guide to Physical Examination and History Taking. 6th ed.* Philadelphia, Pa: JB Lippincott Co; 1991:491-554.

Booher J, Thibodeau G. *Athletic Injury Assessment. 3rd ed.* St. Louis, Mo: Mosby; 1994:88-115, 266-289, 315-353.

Cantu RC. Return to play guidelines after a head injury. *Clin Sports Med.* 1998;17:45-60.

Gennarelli TA. Cerebral concussion and diffuse brain injuries. In: Torg JS, ed. *Athletic Injuries to the Head, Neck, and Face. 2nd ed.* St. Louis, Mo: Mosby-Year Book; 1991:270-282.

Guthkelch AN. Post-traumatic amnesia: Post-concussional symptoms and accident neurosis. *Eur Neurol.* 1980;19:91-102.

Jane JA, Steward O, Gennarelli T. Axonal degeneration induced by experimental noninvasive minor head injury. *J Neurosurg.* 1987;62:96-100.

Lehman LB, Ravich SJ. Closed head injuries in athletes. *Clin Sports Med.* 1990;9:247-261.

Macciocchi SN, Barth JT, Littlefield LM. Outcome after mild head injury. *Clin Sports Med.* 1998;17:27-36.

Price MB, DeVroom HL. A quick and easy guide to neurological assessment. *J Neurosurg Nurs.* 1985;17:313-320.

Saal JA, Sontag MJ. Head injuries in contact sports: Sideline decision making. *Phys Med and Rehab: State of the Art Reviews.* 1987;1:649-656.

Warren WL, Bailes JE. On the field evaluation of athletic head injuries. *Clin Sports Med.* 1998;17:13-26.

CHAPTER 4

Cervical Spine Injuries

Neck injuries are common in people who participate in sporting activities.[1] For the purpose of this chapter, neck injuries will be divided into cervical spine injuries and brachial plexus injuries. While most cervical spine injuries are minor in nature, some can be severe and catastrophic. Cervical spine injuries include minor sprains and strains, sprains with ligamentous instability, disc herniations, fractures, and spinal cord injuries.

There are two algorithms in this chapter. The first is an evaluation of a cervical spine injury. The second is an evaluation of a brachial plexus injury. Ideally, it is best to follow the cervical spine algorithm first in order to rule out a serious cervical spine injury before evaluating for a brachial plexus injury. However, the brachial plexus algorithm does cover the instance when an athlete voluntarily leaves the field of play and approaches the clinician with what initially appears to be an isolated brachial plexus injury. Both algorithms help the clinician to differentiate between a minor cervical sprain, strain, or brachial plexus injury from a more serious cervical spine injury that requires a referral for medical evaluation.

Due to their catastrophic nature, always be prepared for a serious cervical spine injury. It is important to have an ambulance accessible, and hopefully available, at all contests that involve contact sports. Also, it is important to continually practice what to do in the event of a cervical spine injury. Additionally, have access to the proper equipment, including a spine board, tools to remove a facemask, rigid cervical collar, and sandbags to hold the head in place.[2]

There are several ways that the cervical spine can sustain a serious injury. Axial loading of the cervical spine (the neck flexed 30 degrees) is the primary mechanism of injury for severe cervical spine injuries. Other forces, such as hyperflexion, hyperextension, and rotation, may contribute to cervical spine injuries.[2]

It is the primary goal during the initial evaluation and treatment of an athlete with a suspected cervical spine injury to maintain spinal alignment and therefore reduce the chance of a neurological injury occurring. Approximately 50% of individuals with significant spine injuries do not develop neurological signs immediately after the injury has occurred. Therefore, if treated improperly, an athlete with an initially isolated unstable spine injury could be transformed to an athlete with a permanent neurological deficit.[3,4]

Any athlete suspicious of having a neck injury should receive a thorough evaluation for a cervical spine injury. An athlete who has only neck pain or one who has no neck pain and minimal symptoms can still have a significant cervical spine injury. Therefore, evaluation for a possible cervical spine injury should still be performed even if an athlete ambulates to the sideline, complains only of neck pain, and reports no other symptoms.[5,6]

A brachial plexus injury, or "burner," is a temporary dysfunction of the neural structures in the brachial plexus after a blow to the head, neck, or shoulder.[4] The C5 through T1 nerve roots form the complex brachial plexus. After these nerve roots exit the spinal foramen, they reorganize by dividing and combining their sensory and motor components into trunks, divisions, cords, and branches that neurologically supply the upper extremities. While most injuries are isolated to the brachial plexus, the nerve root can be injured.

There are three ways to injure the brachial plexus.[7-9] First, a traction injury can occur in which the ipsilateral shoulder is depressed with concurrent contralateral neck deviation. Traction injuries usually occur in younger athletes (high school age). Although rare in athletics, severe traction of the brachial plexus can cause an avulsion of a nerve root.[10] With a nerve root avulsion, Horner's syndrome may be present (ipsilateral smaller pupil with a drooping eyelid and possible loss of sweating on the ipsilateral forehead).[10] The second mechanism is a compression injury, in which the neck is hyperextended during ipsilateral side bending and/or rotation. Compression injuries commonly occur in older athletes who have some degenerative disc disease and/or foraminal spondylosis (narrowing).[7,9] The third injury to the brachial plexus is a contusion due to a direct blow to the brachial plexus at the supraclavicular or brachial regions. Occasionally, the cervical plexus (C2 to C4) can be affected by the same mechanisms listed above. There is increased risk of developing a brachial plexus compression injury if the clavicle has been fractured and healed with callus formation or if there is a hypertrophic clavicular nonunion. There is also an increased risk of developing a brachial plexus stretch injury if there is glenohumeral instability.[8,10,11]

Brachial plexus injuries commonly occur in rugby, wrestling, ice hockey, and football.[7] One study has shown that 52% of American football players had a brachial plexus injury in one season.[12] American football tackling is a common cause of brachial plexus injuries. Defensive football players, especially linebackers and defensive backs, are most prone to developing a brachial plexus injury.[10]

When evaluating an athlete for a possible brachial plexus injury, the clinician should keep several things in mind. First, the upper trunk of the brachial plexus is most commonly involved. This includes the C5 and C6 nerves. Therefore, the muscles most affected by a brachial plexus injury are the deltoid, external shoulder rotators, and the biceps.[8,13] Second, there is usually a greater motor than sensory loss.[10] A motor deficit may not clinically develop for hours to weeks after the injury. Thus, it is important to re-evaluate athletes for up to 2 weeks after the injury occurs.[10] Third, rotator cuff injuries can also cause weakness in the above muscles. Therefore, tests for tears and/or impingement of the rotator cuff should be performed to rule out concurrent rotator cuff pathology.[8] Fourth, the axillary artery and vein could also be injured during a brachial plexus injury. Therefore, vascular status should be assessed.[10] Fifth, referral should be made to a physician if the symptoms last longer than 1 hour, worsen, or in the event of recurrent injuries.[14] Some clinicians believe that all athletes who develop brachial plexus injuries should be radiographically evaluated.[15]

EVALUATION OF A CERVICAL SPINE INJURY

EMS: Emergency Medical Service.
PRN: As Needed.
*D: Dysfunction-Alert (orientation to person, time and place), responds to Verbal or Painful stimuli, or Unresponsive (AVPU).

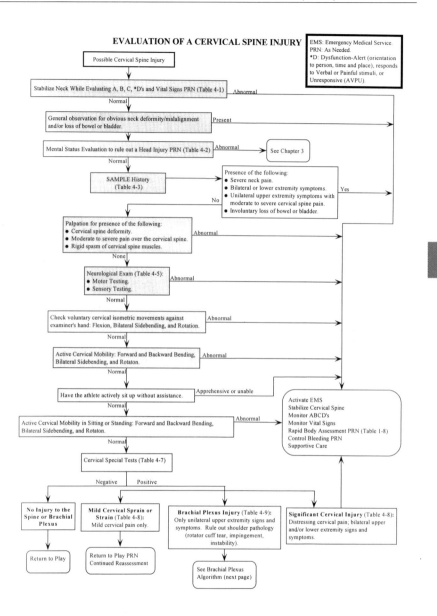

Possible Cervical Spine Injury

Stabilize Neck While Evaluating A, B, C, *D's and Vital Signs PRN (Table 4-1) — Abnormal

Normal

General observation for obvious neck deformity/malalignment and/or loss of bowel or bladder. — Present

Mental Status Evaluation to rule out a Head Injury PRN (Table 4-2) — Abnormal → See Chapter 3

Normal

SAMPLE History (Table 4-3)

Presence of the following:
• Severe neck pain.
• Bilateral or lower extremity symptoms.
• Unilateral upper extremity symptoms with moderate to severe cervical spine pain.
• Involuntary loss of bowel or bladder.
— Yes

No

Palpation for presence of the following:
• Cervical spine deformity.
• Moderate to severe pain over the cervical spine.
• Rigid spasm of cervical spine muscles.
— Abnormal

None

Neurological Exam (Table 4-5):
• Motor Testing.
• Sensory Testing.
— Abnormal

Normal

Check voluntary cervical isometric movements against examiner's hand: Flexion, Bilateral Sidebending, and Rotation. — Abnormal

Normal

Active Cervical Mobility: Forward and Backward Bending, Bilateral Sidebending, and Rotaton. — Abnormal

Normal

Have the athlete actively sit up without assistance. — Apprehensive or unable

Normal

Active Cervical Mobility in Sitting or Standing: Forward and Backward Bending, Bilateral Sidebending, and Rotaton. — Abnormal

Normal

Activate EMS
Stabilize Cervical Spine
Monitor ABCD's
Monitor Vital Signs
Rapid Body Assessment PRN (Table 1-8)
Control Bleeding PRN
Supportive Care

Cervical Special Tests (Table 4-7)

Negative   Positive

No Injury to the Spine or Brachial Plexus

Mild Cervical Sprain or Strain (Table 4-8): Mild cervical pain only.

Brachial Plexus Injury (Table 4-9): Only unilateral upper extremity signs and symptoms. Rule out shoulder pathology (rotator cuff tear, impingement, instability).

Significant Cervical Injury (Table 4-8): Distressing cervical pain; bilateral upper and/or lower extremity signs and symptoms.

Return to Play

Return to Play PRN Continued Reassessment

See Brachial Plexus Algorithm (next page)

EVALUATION OF A BRACHIAL PLEXUS INJURY

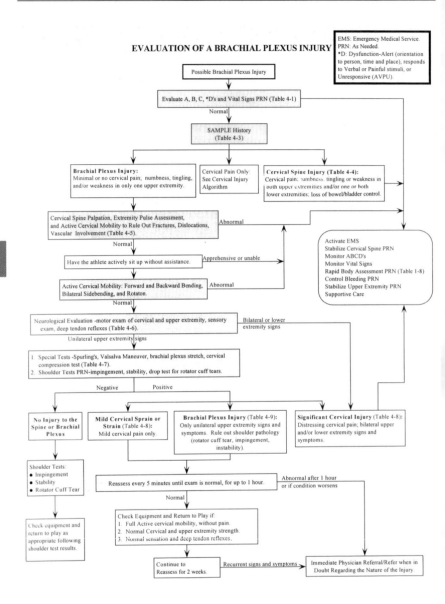

EMS: Emergency Medical Service.
PRN: As Needed.
*D: Dysfunction-Alert (orientation to person, time and place), responds to Verbal or Painful stimuli, or Unresponsive (AVPU).

Possible Brachial Plexus Injury

Evaluate A, B, C, *D's and Vital Signs PRN (Table 4-1)

Normal

SAMPLE History (Table 4-3)

Brachial Plexus Injury: Minimal or no cervical pain; numbness, tingling, and/or weakness in only one upper extremity.

Cervical Pain Only: See Cervical Injury Algorithm

Cervical Spine Injury (Table 4-4): Cervical pain; numbness, tingling or weakness in both upper extremities and/or one or both lower extremities; loss of bowel/bladder control.

Cervical Spine Palpation, Extremity Pulse Assessment, and Active Cervical Mobility to Rule Out Fractures, Dislocations, Vascular Involvement (Table 4-5).

Abnormal

Normal

Have the athlete actively sit up without assistance.

Apprehensive or unable

Active Cervical Mobility: Forward and Backward Bending, Bilateral Sidebending, and Rotation.

Abnormal

Normal

Activate EMS
Stabilize Cervical Spine PRN
Monitor ABCD's
Monitor Vital Signs
Rapid Body Assessment PRN (Table 1-8)
Control Bleeding PRN
Stabilize Upper Extremity PRN
Supportive Care

Neurological Evaluation -motor exam of cervical and upper extremity, sensory exam, deep tendon reflexes (Table 4-6).

Bilateral or lower extremity signs

Unilateral upper extremity signs

1. Special Tests -Spurling's, Valsalva Maneuver, brachial plexus stretch, cervical compression test (Table 4-7).
2. Shoulder Tests PRN-impingement, stability, drop test for rotator cuff tears.

Negative   Positive

No Injury to the Spine or Brachial Plexus

Mild Cervical Sprain or Strain (Table 4-8): Mild cervical pain only.

Brachial Plexus Injury (Table 4-9): Only unilateral upper extremity signs and symptoms. Rule out shoulder pathology (rotator cuff tear; impingement, instability).

Significant Cervical Injury (Table 4-8): Distressing cervical pain; bilateral upper and/or lower extremity signs and symptoms.

Shoulder Tests:
● Impingement
● Stability
● Rotator Cuff Tear

Reassess every 5 minutes until exam is normal, for up to 1 hour.

Abnormal after 1 hour or if condition worsens

Normal

Check equipment and return to play as appropriate following shoulder test results.

Check Equipment and Return to Play if:
1. Full Active cervical mobility, without pain.
2. Normal Cervical and upper extremity strength.
3. Normal sensation and deep tendon reflexes.

Continue to Reassess for 2 weeks.

Recurrent signs and symptoms

Immediate Physician Referral/Refer when in Doubt Regarding the Nature of the Injury.

Table 4-1

Vital Signs: Possible Abnormal Findings in the Presence of a Cervical Spine Injury*

Vital Sign	Abnormal	Interpretations
Pulse	Bradycardia	Possible neurogenic shock
Respiration	Tachypnea; shallow respirations; decreased chest movement and increased abdominal movement	Possible diaphragmatic breathing due to intercostal paralysis
Blood pressure	Decreased	Possible neurogenic shock

*See Table 1-2 for normal data

Table 4-2

Mental Status Evaluation[16,17]

AVPU (alert, responds to verbal or painful stimuli, or unresponsive) as indicated (Table 1-3).
Glasgow Coma Scale as needed and if time permits (Table 1-7).
Orientation to person, time, and place (Table 1-6).
Retrograde amnesia (loss of memory and events that occurred prior to the injury)—
ask the athlete:
*   What do you do on a certain play? (The clinician would need to ask about a specific play.)
*   Do you know what play was run when the injury occurred?
*   Do you know the score of the game?
*   Do you know what team you played in the preceding game?
Post-traumatic amnesia (loss of memory and events that occur after the injury)—
ask the athlete:
*   What do you first recall after the injury?
*   Name four objects and have the athlete repeat them back immediately and 5 minutes later.
Ability to concentrate
*   Name the months of the year backward.
*   Count backward from 100 in multiples of 3.
General impression after the evaluation
*   Facial expression: vacant stare or dazed look.
*   Level of consciousness:
    *   Alert: aware and responds appropriately and quickly to questions asked.
    *   Lethargic: drowsy and falls asleep, but is easily aroused.
    *   Stuporous: asleep most of the time and difficult to arouse; inappropriately responds to verbal stimuli.
    *   Semicomatose: no response to verbal stimuli, but some reflexive response to pain.
    *   Comatose: no response to verbal or painful stimuli; no motor activity.
*   Speech patterns.
*   Emotional state.
*   Appropriate verbal and nonverbal responses to the above questions.

Table 4-3

SAMPLE History

Questions	Interpretation
Symptoms	
Where is the pain located (cervical spine or distal pain)?	Cervical spine pain or cervical spine pain with symptoms radiating to the extremities is indicative of a possible severe cervical spine injury.
Is there any numbness, burning, weakness, and/or tingling present?	These are all symptoms of nerve injury or involvement.
If so, do the symptoms involve the upper and/or lower extremities and are they unilateral or bilateral?	Bilateral or lower extremity symptoms are indicative of a serious cervical spine injury, while unilateral upper extremity symptoms may indicate a cervical spine injury or brachial plexus injury.
Were there any unusual symptoms that occurred during or after the injury, such as snapping, popping, locking, or crepitation?	These are all possible symptoms of a serious cervical spine injury.
Allergies	
Do you have any known allergies?	This information may be helpful to a physician or paramedic.
Medications	
Are you currently taking any medications?	This information may be helpful to a physician or paramedic.
Past Medical History	
Do you have a history of cervical spine trauma or conditions?	The current injury could be an aggravation or progression of a previous injury.
Do you have any congenital anomalies of the spine?	The current injury could be an aggravation or progression of a previous injury.
Do you have a history of shoulder complex injuries or conditions?	Some shoulder injuries can produce signs and symptoms of a cervical injury such as radicular symptoms. An unstable shoulder can place a stretch on the brachial plexus.
Last Meal Eaten	
When was the last time you ate or drank?	This information may be helpful to a physician or paramedic.
Events Leading to the Injury	
Do you know how you were injured?	This may help to differentiate between a possible cervical spine injury and a brachial plexus injury.

Table 4-4

Some Signs and Symptoms of a Significant Cervical Spine Injury[14,18]

- Involuntary loss of bowel and/or bladder control
- Cervical pain without movement
- Pain with palpation over the posterior or anterior cervical spine
- Rigid muscle spasms of the anterior and/or posterior neck muscles
- Deformity detected by palpation or the presence of a wryneck (abnormal neck position usually including flexion, rotation, and side bending)
- Decreased cervical spine mobility with pain
- Persistent burning, weakness, tingling, or numbness in any extremity

Table 4-5
Structures to Palpate During a Brachial Plexus Evaluation

- Cervical spine
- Supraclavicular fossa and axilla
- Clavicle
- Humerus
- Scapula
- Sternum
- Ribs
- Sternoclavicular joint
- Acromioclavicular joint
- Glenohumoral joint
- Distal pulses

Table 4-6
Neurological Evaluation

Nerve	Motor	Sensory	Deep Tendon Reflex
C1	Head and neck flexors	None	None
C2	Head and neck extensors	Top of head	None
C3	Head and neck extensors	Anterior and posterior neck	None
C4	Shoulder shrug	Superior shoulders and chest	None
C5	Shoulder abductors and external rotators	Lateral arm	Biceps
C6	Elbow flexors and wrist extensors	Lateral forearm	Brachioradialis
C7	Elbow extensors and wrist flexors	Middle finger	Triceps
C8	Finger flexors	Medial forearm	None
T1	Finger abductors	Medial arm	None
T12 to L2	Hip flexion	Medial thigh	None
L2 to L4	Knee extension	Anterior thigh	None
L4	Dorsiflexors and inverters	Medial leg	Patella
L5	First toe dorsiflexion	Lateral leg and dorsum of foot	None
S1	Eversion and plantar flexion	Lateral and plantar foot	Achilles

Table 4-7
Cervical Special Tests

Spurling's Test:

The patient extends the head and rotates it toward the injured side while the examiner applies compression to the top of the patient's head. The test is positive if there is an increase in extremity symptoms.

Brachial Plexus Stretch Test:[19]

The examiner depresses the injured shoulder while laterally flexing the head to the contralateral side. The test is positive if there is an increase in upper extremity symptoms.

Valsalva Test:

Sitting, the athlete bears down as if trying to force a bowel movement. The test is positive if there are increased symptoms, indicating injury to the thecal sac (eg, disc herniation).

Compression Test:

The examiner compresses the cervical spine by pushing downward on the athlete's head. The test is positive if there are increased symptoms.

Table 4-8

Cervical Spine Injuries

Condition	Mechanism and General Information	Possible Signs and Symptoms
Cervical strain/mild sprain	1. Caused by neck motion forced beyond normal range or excessive muscle contraction or stretch 2. The most common type of athletic neck injury	1. Point tenderness over the sprain 2. Usually paracervical pain and muscle spasms 3. Loss of cervical motion due to pain and spasms 4. No neurological signs
Cervical spinal cord neuropraxia (transient neurological deficit without nerve degeneration)	1. Caused by contusion of the spinal cord with secondary hemorrhage, edema, and/or ischemia 2. Symptoms depend on the specific aspect of the cord that is injured (the central, anterior, or posterior regions) 3. The most common is burning hands syndrome, which is a form of central cord injury in which the only symptom is burning sensations in both hands 4. May be associated with ligamentous instability, disc pathology, cervical anomalies, or spondylitic changes	1. Usually transient, lasting 15 minutes to 48 hours 2. No neck pain 3. Sensory changes including burning, tingling, and/or numbness 4. Motor changes (can have mild weakness to complete paralysis) 5. Usually bilateral 6. Can affect upper extremities, lower extremities, or both
Cervical instability (grade II or III sprain)	1. Caused by axial compression or hyperflexion disrupting the posterior cervical ligaments 2. May be associated with a fracture and/or dislocation	1. Neck pain at rest and tenderness to palpation 2. Possible step-off with palpation 3. Pain with cervical movement, especially with cervical flexion and extension 4. Neurological deficit (can present with no weakness to complete quadriplegia)
Acute disc herniation	1. Caused by axial compression with a secondary disc fragment or herniation compressing the spinal cord or nerve root 2. May be associated with a fracture and/or dislocation 3. Specific signs and symptoms depend on the level involved	1. Neck pain at rest and tenderness to palpation 2. Decreased cervical spine mobility 3. Unilateral symptoms and signs radiating to the arm are most common. Bilateral involvement of the arms and/or legs is possible 4. Neurological deficits are usually present 5. Nerve root compression will follow dermatomal and myotomal patterns of involvement 6. Usually positive spurling, valsalva, and compression tests
Cervical dislocation (C1-C2 rotary subluxation, unilateral or bilateral facet dislocation)	1. Caused by hyperflexion with rotation 2. Can be unilateral or bilateral 3. Can be stable or unstable 4. May have disc involvement	1. Neck pain at rest and tenderness to palpation 2. Possible step-off noted with palpation 3. Wryneck (abnormal neck position of flexion, rotation, and side bending) 4. Decreased cervical movement due to pain 5. Probable neurological deficits 6. Can cause quadriplegia or sudden death
Cervical spine fractures	1. Primarily caused by axial loading 2. Can be stable or unstable	Same as cervical dislocations

Table 4-9
Brachial Plexus Injuries

Condition	Mechanism and General Information	Possible Signs and Symptoms
Brachial plexus injuries ("burners," or "stingers")	1. Burner: A temporary dysfunction of the neural structures in the brachial plexus after a blow to the head, neck, or shoulder[22] 2. Traction or contusion of the brachial plexus: • Caused by contralateral neck lateral flexion with ipsilateral shoulder depression • Can also be caused by contusion to the brachial plexus due to a blow to the supra-clavicular region	1. No neck pain 2. Normal neck mobility 3. Negative spurling's test 4. Positive brachial plexus stretch test 5. Pain and burning parasthesias from top of shoulder down the arm to the hand 6. The athlete may be holding the arm with the shoulder depressed. 7. Motor weakness, especially with resisted shoulder abduction and external rotation, and elbow flexion 8. No dermatomal pattern of involvement 9. Transient, usually lasting only several minutes
	3. Nerve root compression caused by ipsilateral cervical lateral flexion with extension • Can effect more than one nerve root • Can be isolated to one nerve root	1. Neck pain 2. Decreased neck mobility due to pain 3. Positive spurling's test 4. Negative brachial plexus stretch test 5. If more than one nerve root is involved, (#5-9 above) and symptoms may be present 6. Signs and symptoms may follow the pattern of an isolated nerve root if only one nerve root is involved
	4. Nerve root avulsion	Horner's syndrome (ipsilateral smaller pupil with a drooping eyelid and possible loss of sweating on the ipsilateral forehead)
	5. Rarely, the cervical plexus may be injured	1. Shooting pain to the posterior scalp, behind the ear, around the neck, and/or the top of the shoulder 2. Cervical muscle weakness may occur

References

1. Anderson C. Neck injuries: backboard, bench, or return to play? *Phys Sportsmed.* 1993;21(8):23-34.
2. Posta AG, Clancy WG. Neck trauma. In: Andrews JR, Clancy WG, Whiteside JA, eds. *On-Field Evaluation and Treatment of Common Athletic Injuries.* St. Louis, Mo: Mosby; 1997:97-134.
3. Marks MR, Bell GR, Boumphrey FR. Cervical spine fractures in athletes. *Clin Sportmed.* 1990;9:13-29.
4. Vereschgin KS, Wiens JJ, Fanton GS, Dillingham MF. Burners: don't overlook or underestimate them. *Phys Sportsmed.* 1991;19(9):96-106.
5. Vegso JJ, Torg JS. Field evaluation and management of cervical spine injuries. In: Torg JS, ed. *Athletic Injuries to the Head, Neck, and Face. 2nd ed.* St. Louis, Mo: Mosby-Year Book; 1991:426-437.
6. Warren WL, Bailes JE. On the field evaluation of athletic neck injury. *Clin Sportmed.* 1998;17:99-110.
7. Kelly JD. Brachial plexus injuries: evaluating and treating "burners." *J Musculoskel Med.* 1997;9:70-78.
8. Nissen SJ, Laskowski ER, Rizzo TD. Burner syndrome: recognition and rehabilitation. *Phys Sportsmed.* 1996;24(6):57-64.
9. Torg JS. The cervical spine, spinal cord, and brachial plexus. In: Scuderi G, McCann P, Bruno P, eds. *Sports Medicine: Principles of Primary Care.* St. Louis, Mo: Mosby; 1996:186-201.
10. Hershman EB. Injuries to the brachial plexus. In: Torg JS, ed. *Athletic Injuries to the Head, Neck, and Face. 2nd ed.* St. Louis, Mo: Mosby-Year Book; 1991:338-367.
11. Hershman EB. Brachial plexus injuries. *Clin Sportmed.* 1990;9:311-329.
12. Sallis RE, Jones K, Knopp W. Burners: offensive strategy for an underreported injury. *Phys Sportsmed.* 1992;20(11):47-55.

13. Carter RL, Day AL. Head and neck injuries. In: Mellion M, Walsh W, Shelton G, eds. *The Team Physician's Handbook.* Philadelphia, Pa: Hanley & Belfus; 1990:279-288.
14. Booher J, Thibodeau G. *Athletic Injury Assessment. 3rd ed.* St. Louis, Mo: Mosby; 1994:88-115, 316-353, 563.
15. Gallaspy JB, May JD. *Signs and Symptoms of Athletic Injuries.* St. Louis, Mo: Mosby; 1996:79-100.
16. American Academy of Neurology. Practice parameter: the management of concussion in sports (summary statement). *Neurology.* 1997;48:581-585.
17. Price MB, DeVroom HL. A quick and easy guide to neurological assessment. *J Neurosurg Nurs.* 1985;17:313-320.
18. Torg JS, Ramsey-Emrhein JA. Cervical spine and brachial plexus injuries. *Phys Sportsmed.* 1997;25(7):61-88.
19. Jackson DW, Lohr FJ. Cervical spine injuries. *Clin Sportsmed.* 1986;5:373-386.

Bibliography

Arnheim D. Modern Principles of Athletic Training. St. Louis, Mo: Times Mirror/Mosby College Publishing; 1989:692-733.

Athletic Training Emergency Care. Course Notebook. Wichita, Kan, April 1997 (c/o DCH Outpatient Services, 809 University Boulevard East, Tuscaloosa, AL 35401).

Bailes JE, Maroon JC. Management of cervical spine injuries in athletes. Clin Sportsmed. 1989;8:43-58.

Haynes S. Systematic evaluation of brachial plexus injuries. Athletic Training. 1993;(3)263-267.

Wilberger JE. Athletic spinal cord and spine injuries: guidelines for initial management. Clin Sportsmed. 1998;17:111-120.

Wilberger JE, Maroon JC. Cervical spine injuries in athletes. Phys Sportsmed. 1990;18(3):57-70.

CHAPTER 5

Facial Injuries

Facial injuries can occur in sporting activities from a direct blow to the face by an object or opposing player or from contact with the playing surface. Most facial trauma is minor in nature, such as contusions, mild lacerations, or controllable nose bleeding (epistaxis) and can be treated on the sideline. However, more severe problems, such as moderate to severe lacerations, uncontrollable epistaxis, facial fractures, and injuries to muscles, nerves, and glands can occur and need referral for further medical evaluation. Eye and dental trauma can also occur and are covered in following chapters. The purpose of this chapter is to help the clinician differentiate between relatively mild injuries and more severe injuries.

Always suspect underlying conditions, such as facial fractures or injuries to the muscles, nerves, or glands, in the presence of significant facial contusions or wounds (abrasions, lacerations, puncture wounds). The mechanical structure of the facial bones causes predictable fracture patterns to occur, including fractures of the frontal sinus, orbital blowout, zygoma, nasal, maxillary, and mandibular bones.[1] Also, if epistaxis develops due to trauma, the clinician must first rule out a fracture to the maxillary, zygoma, or nasal bones.[2,3] Facial fractures can be assessed by palpation, bimanual tests, and tests for occlusion. Performing motor and sensory testing of the face can assess for the presence of muscle and nerve injuries. Due to its location, the parotid gland can be easily injured during a facial injury. The parotid gland (a salivary gland) is located inferior to a line from the tragus (the flap of cartilage that is anterior to the external ear opening) to the mouth and posterior to a vertical line intersecting the lateral canthus (the canthi are the corners of the eyes). The parotid duct is located under a line from the parotid gland to the corner of the mouth.[1] If deep lacerations occur over these areas, a gland or duct injury must be suspected.

Skin injuries are a common type of facial injury. When evaluating a facial skin wound, it is important to remember several things. First, wounds to the face can result in massive bleeding due to the high level of blood profusion to the face.[1] Therefore, the amount of bleeding may be out of proportion to the extent of the injury. Second, wounds to the face can be cosmetically serious. Lacerations that are full skin thickness in depth or are located at the eyebrow, canthus, nasolabial fold, corners of the mouth, or perpendicular to facial lines should be treated and closed by a physician. Further, foreign particles (asphalt, gravel, dirt, etc) that are embedded in an abrasion can cause permanent tattooing of the skin. If there is any question regarding the ability to completely remove the foreign particles, a medical referral should be made to scrub the abrasion clean while the skin is anesthetized. However, small lacerations that are partial thickness in skin depth and not located in the areas above can be treated on the sideline.

BRIEF ANATOMY REVIEW

The foundation of the face is composed of a complex set of bones that are connected via sutures. Overlying these bones are several muscles, nerves, glands, and ducts. Please refer to Figures 5-4 and 5-5 on pages 60 and 61 for diagrams.

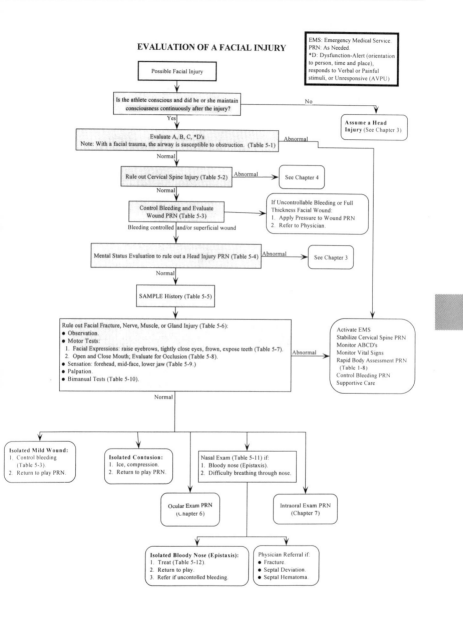

EVALUATION OF A FACIAL INJURY

EMS: Emergency Medical Service.
PRN: As Needed.
*D: Dysfunction-Alert (orientation to person, time and place), responds to Verbal or Painful stimuli, or Unresponsive (AVPU)

Possible Facial Injury

Is the athlete conscious and did he or she maintain consciousness continuously after the injury?

No → **Assume a Head Injury** (See Chapter 3)

Yes

Evaluate A, B, C, *D's
Note: With a facial trauma, the airway is susceptible to obstruction. (Table 5-1)

Abnormal

Normal

Rule out Cervical Spine Injury (Table 5-2) — Abnormal → See Chapter 4

Normal

Control Bleeding and Evaluate Wound PRN (Table 5-3)

If Uncontrollable Bleeding or Full Thickness Facial Wound:
1. Apply Pressure to Wound PRN
2. Refer to Physician.

Bleeding controlled and/or superficial wound

Mental Status Evaluation to rule out a Head Injury PRN (Table 5-4) — Abnormal → See Chapter 3

Normal

SAMPLE History (Table 5-5)

Rule out Facial Fracture, Nerve, Muscle, or Gland Injury (Table 5-6):
• Observation.
• Motor Tests:
  1. Facial Expressions: raise eyebrows, tightly close eyes, frown, expose teeth (Table 5-7).
  2. Open and Close Mouth; Evaluate for Occlusion (Table 5-8).
• Sensation: forehead, mid-face, lower jaw (Table 5-9.)
• Palpation.
• Bimanual Tests (Table 5-10).

Abnormal →

Activate EMS
Stabilize Cervical Spine PRN
Monitor ABCD's
Monitor Vital Signs
Rapid Body Assessment PRN (Table 1-8)
Control Bleeding PRN
Supportive Care

Normal

Isolated Mild Wound:
1. Control bleeding (Table 5-3).
2. Return to play PRN.

Isolated Contusion:
1. Ice, compression.
2. Return to play PRN.

Nasal Exam (Table 5-11) if:
1. Bloody nose (Epistaxis).
2. Difficulty breathing through nose.

Ocular Exam PRN (Chapter 6)

Intraoral Exam PRN (Chapter 7)

Isolated Bloody Nose (Epistaxis):
1. Treat (Table 5-12).
2. Return to play.
3. Refer if uncontolled bleeding.

Physician Referral if:
• Fracture.
• Septal Deviation.
• Septal Hematoma.

Table 5-1

Causes of Airway Obstruction With Facial Trauma

- Tongue occlusion due to central nervous system depression
- Loss of pharyngeal and/or laryngeal reflexes, which allows for aspiration of blood, vomit, foreign bodies (eg, fractured teeth)
- Pharyngeal injury occluding upper airway—can be acute or secondary to swelling of adjacent structures
- Upper airway bleeding
- Profuse tongue or mucosal bleeding
- Posteriorly displaced fractured mandible
- Loosened bridges, dentures, or dislodged or fractured teeth
- An airway obstruction can occur quickly or can develop over a period of time

Table 5-2

Some Signs and Symptoms of a Significant Cervical Spine Injury[4,5]

- Involuntary loss of bowel and/or bladder control
- Cervical pain without movement
- Pain with palpation over the posterior or anterior cervical spine
- Rigid muscle spasms of the anterior and/or posterior neck muscles
- Deformity detected by palpation or the presence of a wryneck (abnormal neck position, usually including flexion, rotation, and side bending)
- Decreased cervical spine mobility with pain
- Persistent burning, weakness, tingling, or numbness in any extremity

Table 5-3

Controlling Facial Wound Bleeding

1. Place the athlete in the sitting or sidelying position to minimize atriovenous pressure
2. Apply direct constant pressure to the wound with a sterile dressing
3. After bleeding has stopped, irrigate the wound with sterile saline
4. Gently debride the wound of any debris
5. Evaluate the extent of the injury
6. If it is a small and partial skin thickness wound, apply an antiseptic ointment (eg, bacitracin or polysporin) and close with sterile strips of tape (eg, Steristrips or butterfly)
7. Cleanse the wound daily with antiseptic soap and water, then redress the wound

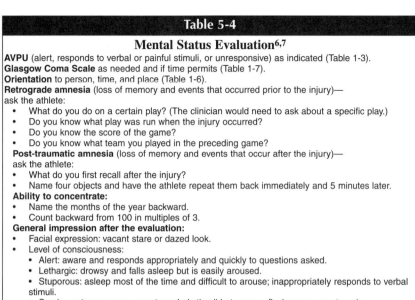

Table 5-4

Mental Status Evaluation[6,7]

AVPU (alert, responds to verbal or painful stimuli, or unresponsive) as indicated (Table 1-3).
Glasgow Coma Scale as needed and if time permits (Table 1-7).
Orientation to person, time, and place (Table 1-6).
Retrograde amnesia (loss of memory and events that occurred prior to the injury)—
ask the athlete:
- What do you do on a certain play? (The clinician would need to ask about a specific play.)
- Do you know what play was run when the injury occurred?
- Do you know the score of the game?
- Do you know what team you played in the preceding game?

Post-traumatic amnesia (loss of memory and events that occur after the injury)—
ask the athlete:
- What do you first recall after the injury?
- Name four objects and have the athlete repeat them back immediately and 5 minutes later.

Ability to concentrate:
- Name the months of the year backward.
- Count backward from 100 in multiples of 3.

General impression after the evaluation:
- Facial expression: vacant stare or dazed look.
- Level of consciousness:
  - Alert: aware and responds appropriately and quickly to questions asked.
  - Lethargic: drowsy and falls asleep but is easily aroused.
  - Stuporous: asleep most of the time and difficult to arouse; inappropriately responds to verbal stimuli.
  - Semicomatose: no response to verbal stimuli but some reflexive response to pain.
  - Comatose: no response to verbal or painful stimuli; no motor activity.
- Speech patterns.
- Emotional state.
- Appropriate verbal and nonverbal responses to the above questions.

Table 5-5

SAMPLE History

Question	Interpretation
Symptoms	
• Where is the pain located?	May identify a possible site of injury
• Can you breathe through your nose?	Nasal involvement
• Are there any visual disturbances?	Possible ocular involvement
• Is there any facial numbness?	Nerve injury
Allergies	
Do you have any known allergies?	This information may be helpful to a physician or paramedic
Medications	
Are you currently taking any medications?	This information may be helpful to a physician or paramedic
Are you currently taking any nonsteroidal anti-inflammatory medications?	These medications could increase intracranial hemorrhaging
Past Medical History	
Have you had any previous facial trauma?	It is not uncommon to have abnormal or asymmetrical facial features prior to the injury. Knowledge of these will help during the evaluation
When was the last tetanus immunization you had? (Note: This question is only important in the presence of a wound)	Tetanus immunizations are effective for 10 years; however, it may be wise for the athlete with a wound to have a "booster" shot if it has been longer than 5 years since the last tetanus shot
Last Meal Consumed	
When was the last time you ate or drank?	This information may be helpful to a physician or paramedic
Events Preceding the Injury	
Do you know how you were injured?	This may help to differentiate between the type of facial injuries the athlete may have

Table 5-6

Some Signs and Symptoms of a Facial Injury Requiring Immediate Medical Referral

Symptom/Sign	Interpretation
Tenderness, crepitation, and/or step-off defect with palpation	Facial fracture
Abnormal shape of face—flattened bones; abnormal shape of the corners of the eyes; elongated, flattened, or C-shaped nose	
Trismus (inability to open the mouth)	
Altered ocular globe (eyeball) position	
Facial numbness	
Diplopia (double vision)	
Diminished eye movements	
Malocclusion	
Deviation with opening of mouth	
Positive bimanual tests	
Hematoma on floor of mouth	
Periorbital ecchymosis	
Ipsilateral narrowed nasal passage	Septal deviation
Bluish bulge that widens nasal septum	Septal hematoma
Uncontrollable nose bleed (epistaxis)	Disruption of posterior nasal vessels or severe disruption of anterior vessels
Deep laceration at site of gland or duct	Suspect gland injury
Muscle weakness or sensation changes	Nerve or muscle injury
Moderate or severe wound	
Significant ocular or intraoral injury (see Chapters 6 and 7)	

Make an immediate medical referral when in doubt regarding the seriousness of the injury

Table 5-7

Motor Tests for Facial Expressions

The only motor nerve to the face is the facial nerve (cranial nerve VII), which has several branches (from superior to inferior):
* The temporal branch innervates the muscles that cause raising of the eyebrows
* The zygomatic and buccal branches innervate the muscles that cause forceful shutting of the eye
* The marginal mandibular branch innervates the muscles that cause smiling
* The cervical branch innervates the platysma, which is used when forcefully showing the lower teeth

Table 5-8

Occlusion[1,8]

1. Ask about the presence of an abnormal occlusion prior to the injury. This can be further clarified by seeing if the wear patterns of the teeth are occlusive with their counterparts.
2. Ask the athlete to close his or her jaws together:
   * The lips and cheeks should be retracted to allow proper viewing of the teeth
   * Normally, the midline of the maxilla and mandible should line up
   * Normally, the first maxillary incisors should slightly override the first mandibular incisors
   * Ask the athlete if he or she perceives the occlusion to be normal
   * Also, if the athlete wears a custom mouth guard, check to see if it still fits properly. If the mouth guard does not fit the way it did prior to the injury, a malocclusion may be present.
3. Palpate over the masseter and temporalis muscles for symmetry of contraction (evaluates motor function of the trigeminal nerve/cranial nerve V)
4. If there is normal occlusion, a maxillary or mandible fracture can usually be ruled out

Table 5-9
Sensation Testing of the Face

Sensation in the face is almost entirely innervated by the three branches of the trigeminal nerve (cranial nerve V):

- The ophthalmic branch innervates the forehead via the supratrochlear and supraorbital cutaneous nerve branches
- The maxillary branch innervates the cheek, upper lip, and nasal skin via the infraorbital cutaneous nerve branch
- The mandibular branch innervates the lower lip and chin via the buccal and mental cutaneous nerve branches

Table 5-10
Bimanual Special Tests to Evaluate Facial Fractures[1,9-11]

1. The examiner stands behind the seated athlete while looking over the top of the athlete's head. The examiner bilaterally places his or her forefingers over anatomical landmarks (infraorbital rims, zygoma) and assesses for symmetry.
2. To assess for a maxillary or mid-face fracture, the examiner places one hand on the athlete's forehead for stabilization. The forefinger and thumb of the other hand are intraorally placed around the anterior maxilla and incisors. The examiner attempts to move the anterior maxilla up and down. The test is positive if movement of the maxilla in up-down and anterior-posterior directions.
3. To assess for a mandibular fracture, the examiner places his or her thumbs bilaterally and intraorally over the mandibular incisors. The examiner's forefingers are placed behind the inferior angle of the mandible. The examiner's other fingers are placed under the inferior mandibular border. The mandibles are then compressed between the thumb and fingers. The examiner, using pressure through the thumbs, attempts to move the teeth medially and laterally, stressing the mandibular arch. The examiner then sequentially places his or her thumbs posteriorly along the molars, stressing the entire arch.

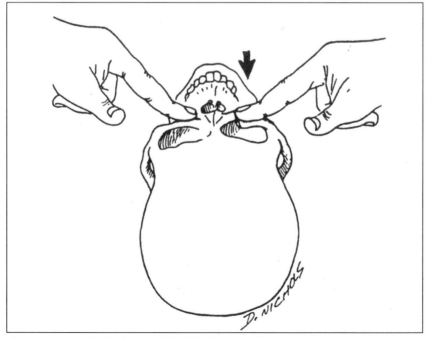

Figure 5-1. Bimanual test for fractures of the infraorbital rims and/or zygoma.

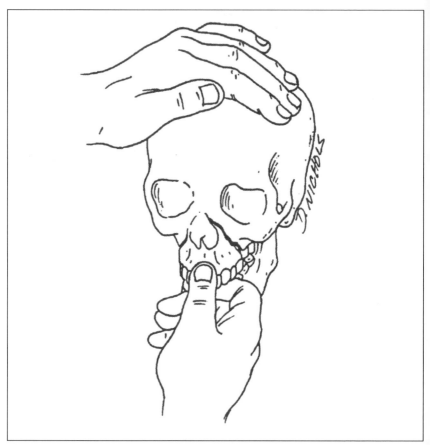

Figure 5-2. Bimanual test for fractures of the maxillary or midface region.

Table 5-11

Nasal Evaluation

External:
- Observation
- Palpation

Internal:
- Requires the use of a pen light and preferably a nasal speculum to spread apart the external nasal opening for proper viewing. The spreading may also be performed manually, but it is difficult.
- Visually assess for the presence of a septal hematoma, septal deviation, foreign body, or the location of profusion in the case of epistaxis.
- Needs to be re-evaluated for several days after traumatic epistaxis due to the possibility of delayed development of a septal hematoma.
- Halo test: collect nasal drainage with a clean gauze pad. If there is a red dot (blood) surrounded by a ring of clear fluid, suspect a cerebrospinal fluid leak.

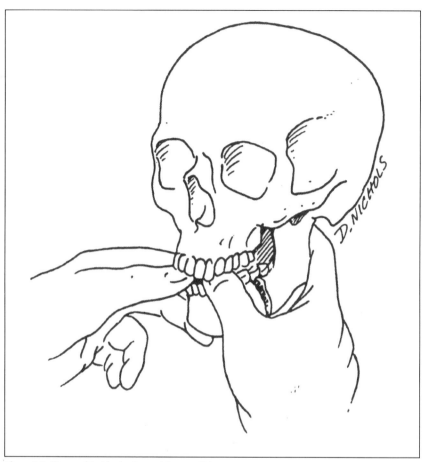

Figure 5-3. Bimanual test for fractures of the mandible.

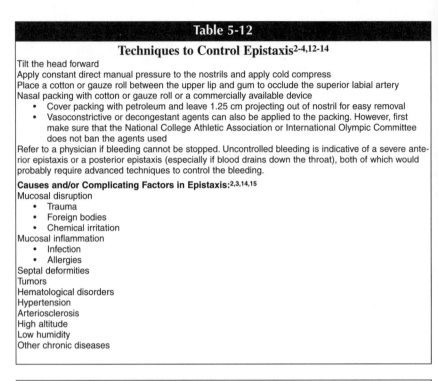

Table 5-12

Techniques to Control Epistaxis[2-4,12-14]

Tilt the head forward
Apply constant direct manual pressure to the nostrils and apply cold compress
Place a cotton or gauze roll between the upper lip and gum to occlude the superior labial artery
Nasal packing with cotton or gauze roll or a commercially available device
- Cover packing with petroleum and leave 1.25 cm projecting out of nostril for easy removal
- Vasoconstrictive or decongestant agents can also be applied to the packing. However, first make sure that the National College Athletic Association or International Olympic Committee does not ban the agents used

Refer to a physician if bleeding cannot be stopped. Uncontrolled bleeding is indicative of a severe anterior epistaxis or a posterior epistaxis (especially if blood drains down the throat), both of which would probably require advanced techniques to control the bleeding.

Causes and/or Complicating Factors in Epistaxis:[2,3,14,15]

Mucosal disruption
- Trauma
- Foreign bodies
- Chemical irritation

Mucosal inflammation
- Infection
- Allergies

Septal deformities
Tumors
Hematological disorders
Hypertension
Arteriosclerosis
High altitude
Low humidity
Other chronic diseases

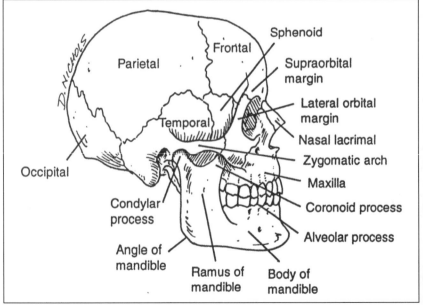

Figure 5-4. Anatomy of the skull.

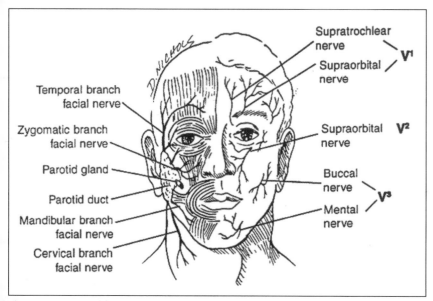

Figure 5-5. Anatomy of the facial nerves and paratid gland.

Table 5-13
Facial Injuries

Condition	Mechanism and General Information	Possible Signs/Symptoms
Frontal sinus fracture	1. Caused by a severe blow to the frontal or supraorbital region 2. Evaluate for cranial or ocular injuries 3. The anterior wall of the frontal sinus is the most commonly fractured site 4. The posterior wall can also be fractured, which requires more force (this rarely occurs)	Anterior wall fracture: 1. Laceration over the supraorbital region—may see bony frag ments 2. Tenderness, crepitation, and/or a step-off defect with palpation 3. Flat appearance of forehead 4. Forehead numbness—sensory nerve injury 5. Edema Posterior wall fracture: 1. Same as above 2. CNS depression 3. Rhinorrhea (fluid loss from the nose) 4. Visible brain matter at laceration site 5. Periorbital ecchymosis 6. Epistaxis (nose bleed) 7. Subconjunctival hemorrhage (blood under conjunctiva)
Zygomatic arch fracture	1. Caused by a severe force applied over the zygomatic arch 2. The bone is usually displaced inferiorly and posteriorly 3. Usually both ends of the arch are fractured	1. Localized edema and ecchymosis 2. Tenderness, crepitation, and/or a central depression defect with palpation 3. Trismus (decreased ability to open the mouth)
Zygomaticomaxillary complex fractures (cheek bone fractures)	1. Caused by a forceful blow to the cheek 2. The bone can be displaced medially, laterally, posteriorly, or inferiorly 3. With displacement, there can be orbital floor or maxillary sinus fractures 4. It is important to evaluate the intraoral and ocular regions	1. Localized edema and ecchymosis 2. Tenderness, crepitation, subcutaneous emphysema, and/or a step-off defect with palpation 3. Appearance of a flattened cheek 4. Trismus 5. Altered globe position, usually inferior 6. Numbness of nose, cheek, and sometimes posterior dental quadrant 7. Impaired upward movement of the eye 8. Diplopia (double vision) 9. Periorbital edema and ecchymosis 10. Lateral subconjuctival hemorrhage 11. Inferior slope of lateral canthus (lateral corner of eye)
Maxilla fracture (le fort fracture or mid-face fracture)	1. Caused by a direct blow with high force 2. The fractured maxilla can be stable or unstable/floating 3. The fractures are rarely symmetrical bilaterally	

Table 5-13, continued

Condition	Mechanism and General Information	Possible Signs/Symptoms
	4. Disruption of the maxillary or paranasal sinuses is possible 5. Airway obstruction can occur due to bleeding or edema of the soft palate	1. Edema and periorbital ecchymosis (raccoon eyes) 2. Tenderness, crepitation, and/or a step-off defect with palpation of the mid face, infraorbital rims, zygomatic arch, and/or superiolateral orbital rim (depends on site of fracture) 3. Appearance of an elongated or flattened face 4. Subcutaneous emphysema over mid-face region 5. Lacerations 6. Malocclusion—open bite deformity (unable to close the front teeth) 7. Numbness of upper lip, cheek, and/or nose 8. Jaw hypomobility 9. Mobile maxilla when tested bimanually 10. Subconjuctival hemorrhage 11. Rhinorrhea
Orbital blowout fracture	Can be isolated or can occur as a component of another facial bone fracture, such as a zygomatic or nasoethmoid fracture	See Chapter 6
Mandible fracture	1. Caused by a direct blow to the mandible 2. The fracture can be single, multiple, fragmented, or avulsed 3. Due to the attachment of the tongue to the anterior mandible; an athlete with a fracture in this area could develop an airway obstruction due to the tongue falling posteriorly 4. A fracture usually extends through the intraoral mucosa 5. Immobilize the athlete with a circumferential bandage (Barton's bandage) that is applied under the chin and over the head	1. Tenderness, crepitation, and/or a step-off defect with palpation 2. Edema and ecchymosis 3. Laceration or abrasion 4. Trismus 5. Malocclusion 6. Deviation with opening of mouth 7. Numbness of lower lip or chin 8. Mobile fragments with bimanual evaluation 9. Dislodged, avulsed, or fractured teeth 10. Gingival lacerations and/or hematoma on floor of mouth
Temperomandibular joint disorders	1. Caused by a blow to the mandible 2. Can cause injuries to the joint capsule, ligaments, meniscus, subluxation, dislocation, or fracture 3. A dislocation or fracture of the mandible can cause difficulty closing the mouth (lockjaw)—an x-ray is needed to differentiate prior to attempts to reduce	1. Decreased mouth opening (normal is 40 mm or the vertical width of three fingers) 2. Lock jaw 3. Deviation to the side of injury with mouth opening 4. Pain and joint noise with opening and biting 5. Malocclusion

Table 5-13, continued

Condition	Mechanism and General Information	Possible Signs/Symptoms
Nasal injuries A. Fractures	1. Caused by a blow to the nose; the nose is more resistant to frontal rather than lateral blows 2. An ocular exam is needed in the presence of a nasal fracture 3. Requires an external and internal nasal evaluation 4. Epistaxis can occur days after the fracture as the swelling decreases	Lateral blow to the nose: 1. C-shaped deformity 2. Usually only involves the nasal bones 3. Epistaxis, usually profuse and self-limiting 4. Swelling 5. Tenderness and crepitation with palpation 6. Increased mobility with medial pressure to the nasal bones 7. Periorbital ecchymosis 8. Nasal airway obstruction Anterior blow to the nose: 1. Flattening or broadening of the nose 2. Fracture may involve the nasoethmoid complex 3. Same as #3 through 8 above 4. Possible cerebrospinal fluid leak from nose 5. Diplopia 6. Traumatic telecanthus (abnormally increased distance between the medial corners of the eyes)
B. Septal deviation	1. Can be dislocated or fractured 2. Usually is associated with a nasal fracture but can occur independently 3. Usually associated with a lateral blow to the nose	1. Nasal airway is obstructed 2. Narrow nasal passage on the ipsilateral side and increased space on the contralateral side
C. Septal hematoma	1. Collection of blood between the septal cartilage and mucous membrane; can lead to the destruction of the nasal septum 2. Requires physician referral for drainage 3. Usually associated with a nasal or septal fracture but can occur independently	1. Requires intranasal evaluation to detect 2. Appears as a bluish bulge that widens the septum 3. Painful to palpation 4. Can be depressed with a cotton-tipped applicator 5. Can develop days after an injury
D. Epistaxis (nose bleed)	1. In athletes, usually occurs due to laceration of the mucosal lining due to trauma or mucosal irritation due to foreign debris (eg. insect) 2. Ninety percent of epistaxis is due to disruption of anterior vessels, while 10% is due to disruption of posterior vessels	The source of anterior epistaxis can usually be seen, primarily drains anteriorly, and is easily controlled. Posterior epistaxis cannot be seen, primarily drains posteriorly down the throat, cannot be stopped with anterior packing, and causes severe bleeding.

References

1. Kaufman BR, Heckler FR. Sports-related facial injuries. *Clin Sports Med.* 1997;16:543-562.
2. Davidson TM. Immediate management of epistaxis. *Phys Sportsmed.* 1996;24(8):74-83.
3. Weir JD. Effective management of epistaxis in athletes. *Athletic Training.* 1997;32:254-255.
4. Booher J, Thibodeau G. *Athletic Injury Assessment. 3rd ed.* St. Louis, Mo: Mosby; 1994:88-115, 290-353.
5. Torg JS, Ramsey-Emrhein JA. Cervical spine and brachial plexus injuries. *Phys Sportsmed.* 1997,25(7):61-88.
6. American Academy of Neurology. Practice parameter: the management of concussion in sports (summary statement). *Neurology.* 1997;48:581-585.
7. Price MB, DeVroom HL. A quick and easy guide to neurological assessment. *J Neurosurg Nurs.* 1985;17:313-320.
8. White MJ, Johnson PC, Heckler FR. Management of maxillofacial and neck soft-tissue injuries. *Clin Sports Med.* 1989;8:11-23.
9. Greenberg AM, Haug RH. Craniofacial injuries. In: Scuderi G, McCann P, Bruno P, eds. *Sports Medicine: Principles of Primary Care.* St. Louis, Mo: Mosby; 1996:129-148.
10. Handler SD. Diagnosis and management of maxillofacial injuries. In: Torg JS, ed. *Athletic Injuries to the Head, Neck, and Face. 2nd ed.* St. Louis, Mo: Mosby; 1991:611-634.
11. MacAfee KA. Immediate care of facial trauma. *Phys Sportsmed.* 1992;20(7):79-91.
12. Arnheim D. *Modern Principles of Athletic Training.* St. Louis, Mo: Times Mirror/Mosby College Publishing; 1989:692-733.
13. Schendel SA. Sports-related nasal injuries. *Phys Sportsmed.* 1990;18:59-74.
14. Stevens H. Epistaxis in the athlete. *Phys Sportsmed.* 1988;16(12):31-40.
15. Viducich RA, Blanda MP, Gerson LW. Posterior epistaxis: clinical features and acute complications. *Ann Emer Med.* 1995;25:592-599.

Bibliography

Carithers JS, Koch BB. Evaluation and management of facial fractures. *Am Fam Phys.* 1997;55:2675-2682.
Colton JJ, Beekhuis GJ. Management of nasal fractures. *Orolaryngol Clin North Am.* 1986;19:73-85.
Crow RW. Sports-related lacerations. *Phys Sportsmed.* 1993;21(2):143-147.
Park SS. Blunt trauma to the face and neck: initial management. *Comp Ther.* 1997;23:730-735.
Tu HK, Davis LF, Nique TA. Maxillofacial injuries. In: Mellion M, Walsh W, Shelton G, eds. *The Team Physician's Handbook.* Philadelphia, Pa: Hanley & Belfus; 1990:302-312.

CHAPTER 6

Eye Injuries

Although the eye is well protected in the skull, it can be easily injured as it naturally turns to look at a potential source of harm or from an unsuspected oncoming projectile.[1,2] While most eye injuries are minor, some serious eye injuries can alter the normal ability of the eye to function. Serious eye injuries can permanently affect vision, which can alter an athlete's performance as well as other aspects of his or her life.[2] This chapter helps the clinician differentiate between a minor eye injury and a more serious one. Minor eye injuries, such as a loose foreign body, periorbital soft tissue contusion, mild lid laceration, or isolated subconjunctival hemorrhage, can be managed on the sideline. However, all other suspected eye injuries should be referred for a medical evaluation.

The eye is divided into two segments: anterior and posterior. The anterior segment is limited anteriorly by the cornea and posteriorly by the iris. Clinically, it includes the iris, pupil, ciliary body, cornea, and anterior aspect of the sclera and conjunctiva. It is filled with a clear fluid called the aqueous humor. The posterior segment is limited anteriorly by the iris and posteriorly by the posterior aspect of the conjunctiva. Clinically, it includes the sclera, choroid, retina, optic nerve, and vitreous humor.

The type of injury an eye receives depends on the mass, size, force, and velocity that the object imparts on the eye.[3] Objects larger than the orbit stress the periorbital structures and possibly the anterior segment. Objects smaller than the orbit cause compression of the eye and anterior or posterior eye segment injuries. Penetrating objects can cause lacerations, abrasions, and/or may pierce the globe. Anterior segment injuries are most common, but posterior segment injuries are associated more with severe injuries that result in vision loss.[4] The most serious eye injuries occur when a superomedially directed force is applied to the inferolateral eye.[5]

Always perform a detailed eye evaluation when an eye injury occurs; a severe eye injury may be present even if the eye appears to look normal.[3] Also, detailed ocular evaluation, assessment, and treatment are important to perform as soon as possible after an eye injury to optimize the visual outcome of the injured athlete.[3,6] An effective ocular evaluation can be performed by taking an accurate history, visual inspection, and the performance of a few simple tests.[7] Additionally, a detailed evaluation should be performed on both eyes after an eye injury.[6]

There are several specific things to keep in mind when evaluating an athlete with a suspected eye injury. First, instruct the athlete not to rub the eyes or tightly close the eyelids (a natural reaction to pain) because this will increase intraocular pressure (IOP), which could cause extrusion of the intraocular contents in the event of a ruptured globe.[2] Second, do not perform an eye evaluation with dirty hands. Preferably, sterile gloves should be worn.[2] Third, do not force the eyelids open to perform an evaluation if they are swollen shut and/or the athlete cannot voluntarily open them. Forcing an exam may make an injury worse, especially if there is a ruptured globe.[7] Fourth, when evaluating an eye injury or when applying gentle pressure to control bleeding, do not place pressure on the globe until a ruptured globe has been ruled out. Fifth, always be aware that multiple eye injuries can be present at one time.

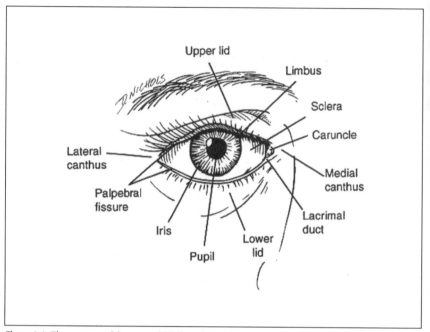

Figure 6-1. The anatomy of the eye and lid (frontal view).

BRIEF ANATOMY REVIEW

Anterior chamber: The space between the iris and cornea that is filled with a clear fluid called the aqueous humor.

Choriod: Blood vessel and connective tissue layer of the eye that lies between the sclera and retina.

Ciliary body: Attaches from the inner eye to the lens and functions to make the aqueous humor, support the lens, and focus the lens.

Conjunctiva: The thin, transparent mucous membrane that covers the inner eyelids and eye. The conjunctiva reflects upon itself to form the inferior and superior fornices, which are recesses between the eyelids and the globe. The aspect of the conjunctiva that covers the eyelids is called the palpebral conjunctiva, and the aspect that covers the eyeball is called the bulbar conjunctiva. It should be noted that the conjunctiva does not cover the cornea.

Cornea: Clear covering in the front of the eye.

Iris: Circular structure that surrounds the pupil and gives the eye its color.

Lens: Sits behind pupil and focuses light on the retina.

Limbus: Junction of the cornea and the sclera.

Macula: Thinnest area of the retina where the sharpest vision occurs, also called the fovea.

Optic nerve: Neural connection between the retina and brain.

Perilimbal area: Area surrounding the cornea.

Periorbita: Area around the eye.

Pupil: Hole in the center of the iris.

Retina: The neurosensory membrane that forms the inner lining of the eye and transforms light to neural impulses.

Sclera: Visible white layer of the eye that covers the eye anteriorly and posteriorly.

Tarsal plates: Located on the posterior aspect of the eyelids, they are firm structures that support the eyelids.

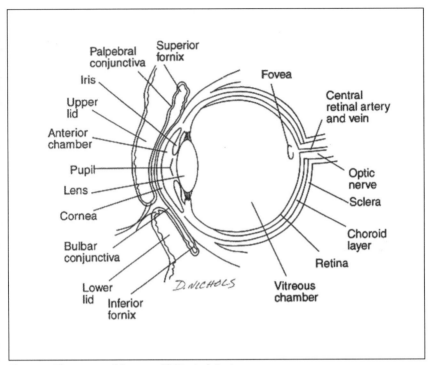

Figure 6-2. The anatomy of the eye and lid (sagittal view).

Uvea: One term used to describe the combination of the iris, ciliary body, and choroid.
Vitreous humor: Clear gel that fills the posterior chamber.
Zonules: Fibers that run radially from the ciliary body to the lens and help to support the lens. The athlete should wear his/her prescription lenses.

EVALUATION OF AN EYE INJURY
(See table 6-1 for needed supplies)

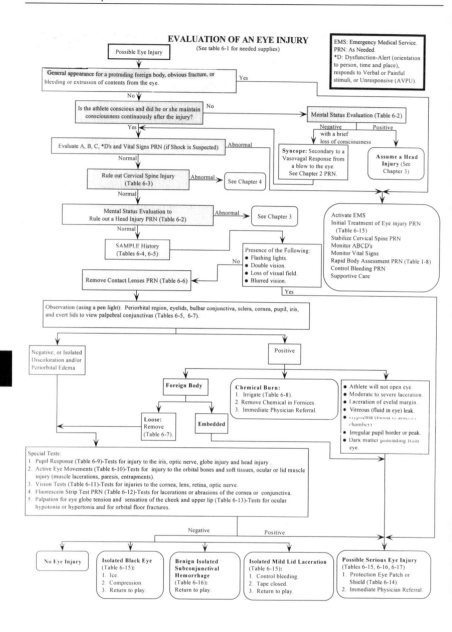

EMS: Emergency Medical Service.
PRN: As Needed.
*D: Dysfunction-Alert (orientation to person, time and place), responds to Verbal or Painful stimuli, or Unresponsive (AVPU).

Possible Eye Injury

General appearance for a protruding foreign body, obvious fracture, or bleeding or extrusion of contents from the eye. — Yes

No

Is the athlete conscious and did he or she maintain consciousness continuously after the injury? — No → Mental Status Evaluation (Table 6-2)

Yes

Negative with a brief loss of consciousness / Positive

Evaluate A, B, C, *D's and Vital Signs PRN (if Shock is Suspected) — Abnormal

Syncope: Secondary to a Vasovagal Response from a blow to the eye. See Chapter 2 PRN.

Assume a Head Injury (See Chapter 3)

Normal

Rule out Cervical Spine Injury (Table 6-3) — Abnormal → See Chapter 4

Normal

Mental Status Evaluation to Rule out a Head Injury PRN (Table 6-2) — Abnormal → See Chapter 3

Normal

SAMPLE History (Tables 6-4, 6-5)

Presence of the Following:
● Flashing lights.
● Double vision.
● Loss of visual field.
● Blurred vision.

No

Remove Contact Lenses PRN (Table 6-6)

Yes

Activate EMS
Initial Treatment of Eye injury PRN (Table 6-15)
Stabilize Cervical Spine PRN
Monitor ABCD's
Monitor Vital Signs
Rapid Body Assessment PRN (Table 1-8)
Control Bleeding PRN
Supportive Care

Observation (using a pen light): Periorbital region, eyelids, bulbar conjunctiva, sclera, cornea, pupil, iris, and evert lids to view palpebral conjunctivas (Tables 6-5, 6-7).

Negative; or Isolated Discoloration and/or Periorbital Edema

Positive

Foreign Body

Chemical Burn:
1. Irrigate (Table 6-8).
2. Remove Chemical in Fornices.
3. Immediate Physician Referral.

● Athlete will not open eye.
● Moderate to severe laceration.
● Laceration of eyelid margin.
● Vitreous (fluid in eye) leak.
● Hyphema (blood in anterior chamber).
● Irregular pupil border or peak.
● Dark matter protruding from eye.

Loose: Remove (Table 6-7).

Embedded

Special Tests:
1. Pupil Response (Table 6-9)-Tests for injury to the iris, optic nerve, globe injury and head injury.
2. Active Eye Movements (Table 6-10)-Tests for injury to the orbital bones and soft tissues, ocular or lid muscle injury (muscle lacerations, paresis, entrapments).
3. Vision Tests (Table 6-11)-Tests for injuries to the cornea, lens, retina, optic nerve.
4. Fluorescein Strip Test PRN (Table 6-12)-Tests for lacerations or abrasions of the cornea or conjunctiva.
5. Palpation for eye globe tension and sensation of the cheek and upper lip (Table 6-13)-Tests for ocular hypotonia or hypertonia and for orbital floor fractures.

Negative / Positive

No Eye Injury

Isolated Black Eye (Table 6-15):
1. Ice.
2. Compression.
3. Return to play.

Benign Isolated Subconjunctival Hemorrhage (Table 6-16):
Return to play.

Isolated Mild Lid Laceration (Table 6-15):
1. Control bleeding.
2. Tape closed.
3. Return to play.

Possible Serious Eye Injury (Tables 6-15, 6-16, 6-17)
1. Protection Eye Patch or Shield (Table 6-14).
2. Immediate Physician Referral.

Table 6-1

Supplies Needed for an Eye Evaluation

- Sterile gloves
- Contact lens suction cup
- Cotton swab
- Pen light
- Eye rinse
- Fluorescein strip
- Eye patch
- Eye shield

Table 6-2

Mental Status Evaluation[8,9]

AVPU (alert, responds to verbal or painful stimuli, or unresponsive) as indicated (Table 1-3).
Glasgow Coma Scale as needed and if time permits (Table 1-7).
Orientation to person, time, and place (Table 1-6).
Retrograde amnesia (loss of memory and events that occurred prior to the injury)—ask the athlete:
- What do you do on a certain play? (The clinician would need to ask about a specific play.)
- Do you know what play was run when the injury occurred?
- Do you know the score of the game?
- Do you know what team you played in the preceding game?

Post-traumatic amnesia (loss of memory and events that occur after the injury)—-ask the athlete:
- What do you first recall after the injury?
- Name four objects and have the athlete repeat them back immediately and 5 minutes later.

Ability to concentrate:
- Name the months of the year backward.
- Count backward from 100 in multiples of 3.

General impression after the evaluation:
- Facial expression: vacant stare or dazed look.
- Level of consciousness:
  - Alert: aware and responds appropriately and quickly to questions asked.
  - Lethargic: drowsy and falls asleep, but is easily aroused.
  - Stuporous: asleep most of the time and difficult to arouse; inappropriately responds to verbal stimuli.
  - Semicomatose: no response to verbal stimuli, but some reflexive response to pain.
  - Comatose: no response to verbal or painful stimuli; no motor activity.
- Speech patterns.
- Emotional state.
- Appropriate verbal and nonverbal responses to the above questions.

Table 6-3

Some Signs and Symptoms of a Significant Cervical Spine Injury[1,6]

- Involuntary loss of bowel and/or bladder control
- Cervical pain without movement
- Pain with palpation over the posterior or anterior cervical spine
- Rigid muscle spasms of the anterior and/or posterior neck muscles
- Deformity detected by palpation or the presence of a wryneck (abnormal neck position usually including flexion, rotation, and side bending)
- Decreased cervical spine mobility with pain
- Persistent burning, weakness, tingling, or numbness in any extremity

Table 6-4
SAMPLE History

Question	Interpretation
Symptoms	
Do you have the feeling that something is in your eye?	Foreign body; abrasion.
Are you experiencing eye pain?	Injury to the eyelid, conjunctiva, cornea, and increased intraocular or intraorbital pressure.
Do you see any mobile or floating spots?	Retinal injury; vitreous detachment or hemorrhage.
Do you see any flashing lights?	Retinal injury.
Are you seeing double? (Note: this question is only valid if the athlete can open both eyes)	Extraocular muscle dysfunction, and orbital fracture; orbital hemorrhage and lens displacement.
Does it seem that a curtain has been lowered over your vision or that you have a loss of your visual field? Or, can you see everything around you?	Narrowed eyelid fissure, corneal opacity, traumatic cataract, vitreous hemorrhage, retinal injury.
Do things look blurry to you?	Optic nerve injury; lens dysfunction, and optic nerve injury; hyphema, vitreous hemorrhage, corneal opacity, traumatic cataract, and retinal injury.
Allergies	
Do you have any known allergies?	A possible cause of conjunctivitis; also, this information may be helpful to a physician or paramedic.
Medications	
Are you currently taking any medications?	Subconjunctival hemorrhage may be caused or increased by taking nonsteroidal anti-inflammatory drugs; also, this information may be helpful to a physician or paramedic.
Past Medical History	
Have you had a recent upper respiratory infection or cold?	Conjunctivitis, which may have been present prior to the current injury.
Have you recently been exposed to pink eye?	Conjunctivitis, which may have been present prior to the current injury.
Do you wear any corrective lenses?	Knowledge of previous visual acuity defects will be helpful during evaluation; inspect glasses for breakage (foreign body, laceration); contact lenses may need to be removed for the evaluation.
Have you had any previous eye disease, injury, or eye surgery?	Previous or current conditions may have a cause or effect on the current eye injury.
Last Meal Consumed	
When was the last time that you ate or drank?	Knowledge may be helpful to a physician or paramedic.
Events Preceding the Injury	
Do you know how you were injured?	Lacerating, scraping, chemical, or concussive injury.
Do you know the size and speed of the object that hit your eye (if applicable)?	Objects smaller then the orbit may cause anterior or posterior segment injuries, while objects larger then the orbit may cause periorbital or anterior segment injuries.

Table 6-5

Some Serious Symptoms and Signs That Require an Immediate Medical Referral

Symptom	Interpretation
Eye pain that is persistent, or eye pain that is moderate or severe in nature	Several possibilities
Foreign body sensation without the appearance of a foreign body	Laceration or abrasion
Perception of mobile spots or floaters in the visual field	Retinal injury
Perception of flashing lights	Retinal injury
Diplopia (double vision)	Orbital wall fracture
Loss of visual field/feeling that a curtain has been pulled over the eye and is blocking vision	Retinal injury
Persistent blurred or impaired vision	Several possibilities
Signs	
Dark tissue protruding through the cornea or sclera	Indicative of a ruptured globe (eyeball)
Hyphema (collection of blood in the anterior chamber)	Several possibilities
Cataract (opacity of lens or its capsule) or loss of corneal clarity	Traumatic cataract or chemical burn
Shallow or protruding anterior chamber	Orbital wall fracture, retrobulbar hemorrhage, lens displacement, or ruptured globe
Pupil distortion, dilation, or constriction	Iritis, optic nerve injury, ruptured globe, or head injury
Irregular pupil or iris shape	Ruptured globe
Pain, photophobia (unusual sensitivity to light), decreased visual acuity, conjunctiva hypermia (redness), and chemosis (edema)	Chemical or radiation burns
Restriction of eye movements	Orbital wall fracture, retrobulbar hemorrhage
Vitreous leak	Ruptured globe
Loss of visual acuity or peripheral vision	Injuries to cornea, lens, retina, or optic nerve
Palpable defect of the orbital rims or periocular area	Orbital wall or rim fracture
Inability of the athlete to actively open eye for examination	Several possibilities
Photophobia	Several possibilities
Afferent pupil defect	Ruptured globe, retrobulbar hemorrhage, or optic nerve injury
Scotoma (blind spot perceived by the athlete) in the central visual region	Optic nerve injury
Lacerations of the lids that are moderate or severe, full thickness lacerations, lid margin lacerations	Suspected abrasion or laceration of the eye surface

Make an immediate medical referral whenever in doubt regarding the seriousness of the injury

Table 6-6

Contact Lens Manipulation[7]

Reposition of a Displaced Lens:
1. Have the athlete try to do it him- or herself
2. Examiner can reposition the lens indirectly through manipulation of the eyelid
3. A hard lens can be repositioned via the use of a contact lens suction cup

A Contact Lens Should be Removed if the Wearer Has Pain or Discomfort:
1. Have the athlete try to remove the lens him- or herself
2. Soft lens: have the athlete look up, which will cause the lens to partially drop onto the lower aspect of the eye. Place finger on the inferior aspect of the lens and maneuver the lens to the lower fornix. Pinch the lens between two fingers and remove it.
3. Hard lens: have the athlete open the eye widely. Grasp the lateral canthus and pull it laterally. Then ask the athlete to forcefully blink. The lens should pop out.

Table 6-7

Eversion of Eyelid for Inspection or Removal of Foreign Body[1,12,13]

Lid eversion should not be performed if a ruptured or perforated globe is suspected.

The simplest way to look for a foreign body is to have the athlete look in all directions as the examiner tries to see if a foreign body is present.

Upper Lid

The examiner asks the athlete to look downward. The examiner then grasps the upper lid and pulls it away from the eye. A cotton swab is then pushed downward on the superior aspect of the upper lid while the upper lid is pulled over the swab, backward toward the eyebrow. If a foreign body is found, it can be removed with a moist sterile cotton swab. The athlete should be instructed to continue to look downward. The cornea should not be touched, as this will cause the athlete to naturally pull away and look upward.

Lower Lid

Have the athlete look upward. The examiner gently places a finger over the lower lid. The lid is pulled downward, exposing the lower fornix. A foreign body is removed as above, using a moist cotton swab while the athlete looks upward.

If the foreign body is embedded in the eye, do not remove the object. Place a shield over the eye and refer the athlete to a physician.

Table 6-8

Chemical Burn Treatment[12]

1. Immediately flush the eye with several liters of fluid for 15 to 20 minutes.
2. Preferably use eye rinse, sterile saline, or Ringer's lactate. Tap water can be used if these fluids are not available.
3. Preferably, flush with a stream of fluid by using a squeeze bottle, eye rinse sink, or intravenous tubing connected to the bag of fluid.
4. Stream the fluid on the sclera so that it can flow over the cornea. Direct streaming on the cornea could cause an abrasion.
5. Evert the eyelids and flush the fornices.
6. Remove remaining chemical matter with a cotton swab as mentioned in Table 6-7.
7. Repeat flushing the eye as stated in #1 above.
8. Immediate referral to a physician is required after flushing the eye.

Table 6-9

Pupil Response Tests*[6,12,14]

Pupil Reactivity Test

1. Preferably done with the lights dim.
2. Have the athlete look into the distance.
3. Shine a bright light into one eye and monitor how quickly the pupil constricts and its size.
4. Repeat the test on the other side and compare the pupils' reaction time and size of constriction.

Swinging Flashlight Test: Tests for the presence of an afferent pupillary defect (optic nerve damage).

1. Normally, there should be a consensual response so that a reactive constriction of one pupil will cause a constriction of the other pupil.
2. Have the athlete look into the distance and test the pupil for its reaction to light as described above.
3. Shine the light for 3 seconds.
4. Quickly shine the light on the other eye for 3 seconds. The eye should already be fully constricted.
5. Then, quickly shine the light again on the first pupil. It should also be fully constricted and thus no movement should be noticed.
6. The test is abnormal if the pupil dilates or if it further constricts (it should already be fully constricted).

*Tests for Iris, optic nerve, globe, and head injuries

Table 6-10
Active Eye Movements*

Do not test for active eye movements if a ruptured or perforated globe is suspected.

Eyelid Movements

Have the athlete try to fully open and close the eyelids.

Extraocular Eye Movements

1. Have the athlete look in all directions—up, down, medially, laterally, and in all four quadrants.
2. Evaluate for any restrictions or limitations in the quantity of movement.
3. Ask the athlete if he or she notices any visual changes, especially double vision, when gazing in different directions.

*Tests for injuries to the orbital bones and soft tissues, or ocular or lid muscles, including muscle lacerations, paresis, and entrapments[2,3,13,14]

Table 6-11
Vision Tests*

Visual Acuity

1. Have the athlete wear his or her corrective lenses if applicable.
2. If his or her corrective lenses are not available, use over-the-counter reading glasses or have the athlete look through a pinhole in a card.
3. Test both eyes, one at a time. Cover the eye not being tested.
4. Have the athlete read the smallest line possible on the near card (Figure 6-3) or have the athlete read different-sized print from a program or newspaper.
5. If the athlete cannot read the card, test for the ability to count fingers at different distances.
6. If the athlete cannot count fingers, test for the ability to detect light perception (use a flashlight) at different distances.

Confrontational Visual Field Test for Peripheral Vision

1. The examiner stands 3 feet in front of the athlete.
2. The athlete covers the nontested eye with his or her hand. The examiner covers his or her opposite eye with a hand. (If the athlete's left eye is being tested, the athlete covers the right eye. The examiner faces the athlete and covers his or her own left eye so that the athlete's and examiner's open eyes are facing each other.)
3. The examiner makes a fist and places it off to one side. The examiner raises some fingers and then closes his or her fist. The athlete is asked to determine the number of fingers that were held up. The examiner repeats this at different distances and all around a horizontal clock at the level of the eye.
4. The examiner compares the range of his or her peripheral vision with that of the athlete's. Repeat with the other eye.

*Tests for injuries to the cornea, lens, retina, and optic nerve[2,6,12]

Table 6-12
Fluorescein Tests*

Fluorescein Strip Test

1. Moisten the fluorescein strip with water.
2. Touch the strip to the inner aspect of the athlete's lower lid.
3. Have the athlete blink a few times to spread the green dye over the eye.
4. Any abrasions or lacerations will appear as bright green.
5. The bright green stain can be more easily seen with a blue-filtered light.

Seidel Test: Tests for a corneal perforation with clear aqueous humor leak.

1. Hold a dry fluorescein strip just below the area of the possible perforation and leak.
2. If a leak is present, the fluid will flow onto the strip.
3. Green dye will appear to run down the eye below the test strip.

*Tests for lacerations or abrasions of the cornea or conjunctiva[1,7,12,15]

Table 6-13

Palpation[12,14]

Do not test for active eye movements if a ruptured or perforated globe is suspected.

Orbital Palpation

Palpate the orbital rims and periorbital region for tenderness, step-off defects, and/or subcutaneous emphysema (a subcutaneous crackling sensation to palpation due to an air collection in the soft tissues).

Ocular Pressure

1. Gently press on the bilateral anterior globes with the eyes closed.
2. Compare the firmness to the eyes bilaterally, as well as to the examiner's own eyes.
   - Ocular hypertonia (increased IOP and firmness): glaucoma, retrobulbar hemorrhage, orbital edema
   - Ocular hypotonia (decreased IOP and firmness): ruptured globe

Sensation Testing of the Face to Rule out a Facial Fracture or Nerve Injury

Evaluate for sensation over the forehead, check, upper lip, and chin (Table 5-9).

Table 6-14

Initial Management of Suspected Serious Eye Injuries[2,4,6]

Apply an Eye Patch if an Isolated Abrasion or Laceration of the Cornea or Conjunctiva has Occurred

1. Have the patient close his or her eyes.
2. Fold an eye patch in half and place it over the injured eye.
3. Place a second eye patch (unfolded) over the first patch.
4. Place tape over the patches to secure them in place.

Apply an Eye Shield Over the Eye For All Other Injuries

1. Place a commercially available eye shield over the eye. If not available, use the bottom of a cup or the lid of a jar. Make sure that the shield is placing pressure on the orbital bones and not on the globe.
2. Tape the shield in place.
3. Ideally, it is best to shield both eyes in order to diminish eye movement.

Calm the athlete and keep him or her quiet in order to minimize exertion.
Try to keep the head elevated 45 degrees while he or she is transported to the hospital.
Do not allow the athlete to eat or drink in order for preparation of possible surgery.

Table 6-15

Periorbital Injuries

Condition	Mechanism and General Information	Possible Signs/Symptoms
Periorbital ecchymosis (black eye)	1. Caused by blunt trauma to the periorbital region. 2. Blood from injured tissues fills the subcutaneous tissues around eye. 3. May be associated with severe injuries to the globe or facial fractures. 4. Do not force the lids open if the athlete cannot voluntarily open them for the eye evaluation; this may cause an expulsion of intraocular contents if the globe is ruptured.	1. Black eye 2. Localized pain 3. Edema may restrict lid movement
Lid laceration	1. May be caused by blunt, sharp, penetrating, and/or projectile trauma. 2. May be associated with an eye abrasion, laceration, or globe injury. Therefore, all lid injuries require a complete eye evaluation. 3. An injury may appear to be externally mild, while it actually caused severe damage to retro lid surface and/or lid muscle. The evaluation should include lid eversion and testing lid opening and closing. 4. Serious lacerations include full skin thickness injuries, lacerations of lid margins, tarsal plate injuries, ptosis, and decreased eye or lid movement. 5. Isolated mild lid lacerations of partial skin thickness can be treated by the PT/ATC with gentle tamponade and sterile taping. The eye should not be covered in order to continually assess any vision changes that would require medical referral.	1. Obvious laceration and external bleeding 2. Damage may be subtle
Injury to lacrimal drainage system	1. Caused by trauma to the medial canalicular region. 2. May be difficult to assess secondary to soft tissue swelling.	1. Excessive tearing 2. Laceration between the medial canaliculus (corner of eye) and nose 3. Laceration of the medial upper or lower lid
Medial wall fracture	1. Caused by blunt force to the anterior orbit. 2. Often, there is a communication between the orbit and ethmoid sinus causing air to leak out of the sinus, leading to subcutaneous emphysema. This is manifested as a subcutaneous crackling sensation during palpation.	1. Pain 2. Binocular diplopia (double vision) in any field of gaze 3. Swelling and ecchymosis of eyelics 4. Enophthalmos (posterior displacement of globe with a sunken in appearance and possible ptosis/drooping eyelid) 5. Subcutaneous emphysema (a subcutaneous crackling sensation with palpation due to air collection in the soft tissues) 6. Palpable step-off defect at orbital rim

Table 6-15, continued

Condition	Mechanism and General Information	Possible Signs/Symptoms
Orbital floor fractures	1. Also caused by blunt force to the anterior orbit. 2. Associated with other eye injuries. 3. Commonly, there is entrapment of the inferior rectus muscle, cranial nerve III damage, and/or scarring of the eye tissue to the fracture. 4. With orbital blowout injuries, the medial orbital wall and orbital floor are most commonly fractured since they are the thinnest bones that make up the bony ocular orbit.	1. Pain 2. Binocular diplopia, especially with upward gaze 3. Swelling and ecchymosis of eyelids 4. Enophthalmos 5. Palpable step-off defect at orbital rim 6. Restricted eye movement, especially upward movement 7. Inferior displacement of globe 8. Numbness over cheek, upper lip, and upper gum and teeth
Retrobulbar hemorrhage	1. Bleeding in posterior orbit behind eyeball. 2. Bleeding may be due to fractured orbital bones, globe injuries, or trauma of the orbital vessels (eg, deep laceration around eyelid). 3. The bleeding may be acute or delayed.	1. Exophthalmos (eye appears to be bulging outward) 2. Corneal exposure 3. Increasing pain and decreasing vision 4. Decreased eye movements 5. Increased IOP 6. Diplopia (double vision) 7. Subcutaneous hemorrhage 8. Afferent pupil defect 9. Conjunctival chemosis (edema/swelling of the conjunctiva) 10. Loss of parallel alignment of eyes

Table 6-16

Anterior Segment Injuries

Condition	Mechanism and General Information	Possible Signs/Symptoms
Foreign bodies (conjunctival and corneal)	1. Commonly caused by track cinders, dirt, or glass 2. Tears usually flush out the object. 3. Evaluation includes eversion of the upper and lower lids to examine the conjunctival fornices, especially when there are vertical abrasions on the conjunctiva or cornea.	1. Sensation of something in the eye 2. Pain 3. Irritation, especially with blinking 4. Tearing 5. Localized hyperemia (redness) 6. Papillary reaction (small bumps) on conjunctiva 7. Possible decreased vision when on the cornea
Lacerations and abrasions (cornea, conjunctiva, and sclera)	1. Trauma from scraping and wiping of sharp objects such as fingernails, broken glass, cinders, etc. 2. There could be an underlying penetrating injury with a globe rupture. Penetration usually occurs near or through the cornea. 3. Evaluate for the presence of a foreign body. If a laceration occurs with the foreign body still in the eye, patch the eye and refer to a physician with the foreign body in place. 4. When evaluating the eye, avoid pressure on the globe until a globe rupture has been ruled out. 5. The injury can be confirmed with the fluorescein dye test. 6. The sclera is too tough to become abraded, but it can be lacerated with a deep conjunctival laceration. 7. Contact lenses should be removed, as they can cause an abrasion to develop into an ulcer. 8. A pressure patch should be applied. However, if a globe injury is suspected, a protective shield should be used instead.	1. Extreme pain 2. Sensation of foreign body in the eye 3. Epiphora (excessive tearing) 4. Gritty sensation 5. Photophobia (abnormal sensitivity to light) 6. Conjunctival chemosis (swelling or edema) 7. Conjunctival hyperemia (redness) 8. Lid laceration 9. Eyelid edema 10. Decreased vision if cornea is involved 11. Subconjunctival hemorrhage 12. If there is a presence of a reddish brown or dark blue material protruding through the laceration, it is the uvea. This is a sign of a globe rupture.
Traumatic iritis	1. Inflammation of the iris and ciliary body. 2. Caused by blunt trauma to the eye.	1. Pain 2. Photophobia 3. Tearing 4. Miosis (small pupil), difficulty with pupil dilatation 5. May have mydriasis (dilated pupil) due to damage of iris sphincter 6. Cloudy anterior chamber with blurred or decreased vision 7. Irregular shape of the iris or pupil 8. Hyperemia (redness) in the perilimbal area
Hyphema	1. Accumulation of blood in the anterior chamber of the eye, anterior to the iris and posterior to the cornea. 2. Caused by blunt trauma to the eye, which ruptures arterioles.	1. Red fluid layer in the anterior chamber 2. Decreased view of the iris and sometimes the pupil 3. Pain

Table 6-16, continued

Condition	Mechanism and General Information	Possible Signs/Symptoms
	3. Begins with a red tinge, but the blood settles inferiorly over a few hours. 4. Associated with orbital fractures, separation of the iris and ciliary body, vitreous hemorrhage, posterior eye injuries, retinal detachments, and sclera rupture. 5. Rebleeding occurs in 10% to 20% of patients over the following 1 to 5 days.	4. Photophobia 5. Decreased vision 6. May be drowsy (unknown mechanism) 7. May be asymptomatic
Chemical burns	1. Commonly caused by irritation from pool chemicals or lime (used to line fields). 2. Requires copious irrigation of the eye for 20 to 30 minutes prior to emergency referral. 3. Remove chemical that may be matted under the eyelids	1. Pain 2. Burning 3. Photophobia 4. Visual loss 5. Conjunctiva hyperemia (redness) and chemosis (edema) 6. Cornea can be abraded, cloudy, or opaque
with a cotton swab. Radiation burns	1. Excessive radiation (sunlight) exposure. 2. Usually there is a delayed onset of symptoms.	1. Pain 2. Photophobia 3. Decreased visual acuity 4. Fluorescein dye test shows scattered areas of defects on the corneal surface
Traumatic cataract and lens displacement	1. Caused by blunt or perforating injuries to the lens.	Traumatic cataract (opacity of the lens or its capsule): 1. Anterior opacity 2. Blurred vision Lens dislocation or subluxation: 1. Irregular depth of anterior chamber 2. Vitreous in anterior chamber 3. Blurred or decreased vision 4. See lens borrowed in anterior chamber or vitreous 5. Monocular diplopia
Dislodged contact lens	1. Lens becomes dislodged off of cornea onto conjunctiva. 2. More common with hard vs. soft lenses.	1. Impaired vision 2. Foreign body sensation 3. Athlete can usually identify the problem

Subconjunctival hemorrhage	1. Hemorrhage under the conjunctiva. Obscures sclera but not the cornea, iris, or pupil.
	2. Causes:
	  a. Trauma: blunt injury or laceration
	  b. Spontaneous
	  c. Valsalva maneuver: strain, weightlifting, vomit
	  d. Conjunctivitis: bacterial, viral, or allergies
	3. Can be benign or serious.
		Benign: no other signs or symptoms; painless and localized conjunctivitis:
		1. Burning, itching, tearing; may have fever
		2. Edema of lids and periorbital skin
		3. Discharge from the eye (ropy, serous, or mucoid)
		4. May have bilateral eye redness
		Severe underlying injury:
		Blurred or decreased vision; pain; decreased eye movement; hyphema; conjunctival chemosis; lid swelling; pupil or

Table 6-17

Posterior Segment Injuries

Condition	Mechanism and General Information	Possible Signs/Symptoms
Retinal edema	1. May be caused by blunt trauma, exercising in high altitude (mountain climbing), or valsalva maneuver (weight training). 2. Can lead to the development of retinal holes or detachment. 3. Associated with retinal hemorrhage and choroid rupture.	1. Can be asymptomatic if it occurs at the periphery of the retina 2. Can have blurred or distorted vision if it occurs at the macula 3. Can have rapid deterioration of visual acuity
Retinal breaks	1. Caused by blunt trauma. 2. There can be a delayed onset of symptoms.	1. Floaters (complaints of black dots, dust, or smoke) if there is a peripheral tear 2. Complaints of flashing lights 3. Profound loss of central vision (central scotoma) if tear occurs in the macula 4. May be asymptomatic
Retinal detachment	1. Caused by blunt trauma. 2. Fluid seeps into the retinal break and separates the neurosensory tissue from its connective tissue. 3. Test visual acuity and visual field.	Macular involvement: 1. Severe loss of central vision Peripheral involvement: 1. Light flashes 2. Floaters 3. Visual field defect; complaint of "curtain coming down" into field of vision
Choroid rupture	Caused by blunt trauma that breaks the choroid and damages the retina, which causes retinal or vitreous hemorrhage.	Decreased peripheral vision (peripheral damage) or central vision (macula damage)
Vitreous hemorrhage	Caused by blunt trauma that leads to hemorrhage from the choroid or retina.	1. Presence of floaters 2. May significantly decrease vision
Ruptured globe	1. Blunt trauma to the eye with an object smaller than the size of the orbit. A rupture of the sclera occurs, usually at its thinnest aspect, which is beneath the insertion of the rectus muscle. Therefore, it is not directly visible. 2. A ruptured globe can also occur at the anterior eye segment due to a penetrating injury at or near the cornea. 3. A loss of intraocular contents usually occurs.	1. Visual protrusion of uvea (dark substance) or vitreous fluid 2. Decreased eye movements 3. Hyphema and/or blood in eye cavities 4. Conjunctival chemosis and/or hyperemia 5. Hypotonia of eye with secondary deep anterior chamber 6. Pain and visual loss 7. Afferent pupillary defect 8. Irregular pupil shape (beaked)—iris pulled toward rupture 9. Subconjunctival hemorrhage
Optic nerve injury	Caused by severe blunt trauma.	1. Afferent pupilary defect 2. Central scotoma (blind spot in central vision)

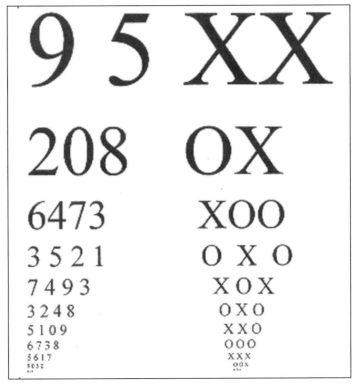

Figure 6-3. Near card. Hold this card 14 inches from the eye in good light. Test each eye separately. The athlete should wear his or her prescription lenses.

References

1. Easterbrook M, Johnston RH, Howcroft MJ. Assessment and management of ocular foreign bodies. *Phys Sportsmed.* 1997;25(2):77-87.
2. Kunh F, Witherspoon CD, Morris R, Kaiser G. Ocular and periocular trauma. In: Andrews JR, Clancy WG, Whiteside JA, eds. *On-Field Evaluation and Treatment of Common Athletic Injuries.* St. Louis, Mo: Mosby; 1997:16-29.
3. Erie JC. Eye injuries: prevention, evaluation, and treatment. *Phys Sportsmed.* 1991;19(11):108-120.
4. Skolik SA, Alfaro DV, Liggett PE. Posterior segment injuries. In: Zaglebaum BM, ed. *Sports Ophthalmology.* Cambridge, Ma0: Blackwell Science; 1996:210-223.
5. Biesman BS, HornblassA. Anatomy. In: Zaglebaum BM, ed. *Sports Ophthalmology.* Cambridge, MA: Blackwell Science; 1996:154-183.
6. Grewal RK, Dhaliwal DK, Hersh PS, Zagelbaum BM. Anterior segment injuries. In: Zagelbaum BM, ed. *Sports Ophthalmology.* Cambridge, MA: Blackwell Science; 1996:184-209.
7. Brucker AJ, Kozart DM, Nichols CW, Raber IM. Diagnosis and management of injuries to the eye and orbit. In: Torg JS, ed. *Athletic Injuries to the Head, Neck, and Face. 2nd ed.* St. Louis, Mo: Mosby-Year Book; 1991: 305-322.
8. American Academy of Neurology. Practice parameter: the management of concussion in sports (summary statement). *Neurology.* 1997;48:581-585.
9. Price MB, DeVroom HL. A quick and easy guide to neurological assessment. *J Neurosurg Nurs.* 1985;17:313-320.
10. Booher J, Thibodeau G. *Athletic Injury Assessment. 3rd ed.* St. Louis, Mo: Mosby; 1994: 88-115, 316-353.
11. Torg JS, Ramsey-Emrhein JA. Cervical spine and brachial plexus injuries. *Phys Sportsmed.* 1997;25 (7):61-88.
12. Mendelsohn M, Abramson D. Eye injuries. In: Scuderi G, McCann P, Bruno P, eds. *Sports Medicine: Principles of Primary Care.* St Louis, Mo: Mosby;1996:115-128.

13. Zagelbaum BM. Sport-related eye trauma: managing common injuries. *Phys Sportsmed.* 1993;21(9):25-40.
14. Christensen GR. Eye injuries in sport: evaluation, management, and prevention. In: Mellion M, Walsh W, Shelton, G eds. *The Team Physician's Handbook.* Philadelphia, Pa: Hanley & Belfus;1990:289-301.
15. Zagelbaum BM. Treating corneal abrasions and lacerations. *Phys Sportsmed.* 1997;25(3):38-44.

Bibliography

Zagelbaum BM, Hochman MA. A close look at a "red eye": diagnosing vision-threatening causes. *Phys Sportsmed.* 1995;23(11):85-92.
Zagelbaum BM, Hochman MA. Examining a "red eye": diagnosing non-vision-threatening causes. *Phys Sportsmed.* 1995;23(12):56-64.

CHAPTER 7

Dental Injuries

Dental trauma due to sports participation has decreased in recent years due to the use of mouth guards and facial shields. However, dental injuries still occur, especially in sports in which mouth guards and facial shields are not mandatory.[1] Dental injuries can be mild, moderate, or severe in nature. The purpose of this chapter's algorithm is to help the clinician differentiate between the types of dental injuries. A mild dental injury includes a partial mucosal thickness laceration and can be managed at the sideline. Moderate dental injuries include a class I or II crown fracture or a nondisplaced tooth injury. Athletes with moderate injuries can continue to play but should be referred to a dentist after the game or contest. Severe injuries include a class III crown fracture, root fractures, alveolar bone fracture, a tooth displacement, or a full thickness mucosal laceration. All severe injuries need an immediate referral to a dentist.

There are three basic mechanisms of tooth injuries.[2] First is a high-velocity direct force, which usually fractures teeth (a direct blow to a tooth, especially the anterior maxillary teeth). The second is a low-velocity direct force (force cushioned by the lips or cheek). This usually causes a tooth displacement. Posterior teeth have more root stability; therefore, anterior teeth are more susceptible to root displacement injuries.[3] Also remember that when a tooth is displaced, there is usually an injury to the periodontal ligament.[3] The third mechanism of a tooth injury is an indirect force, such as the mandible colliding with the maxilla. This can cause posterior tooth injuries. All types of traumatic tooth injuries are often accompanied by soft tissue injuries including hemorrhage, swelling, and lacerations.[3] Also, all traumatic dental injuries, even without obvious injury, can cause damage to the pulp.[4]

It is best to wear sterile gloves when performing an intraoral evaluation. Keep in mind the underlying artery, vein, and nerve structures when performing the evaluation. Also, the lingual and submandibular glands and ducts are located under the floor of the mouth. The parotid gland is located lateral to the second maxillary molars.[3] All of the above can be injured in a dental trauma. Carefully inspect for a laceration of the intraoral mucosa. Intraoral lacerations that extend beyond the mucosa lining need to be referred for suturing. Primary healing without appropriate suturing could lead to a contracture, which would affect the cosmetic and/or functional outcome.[5] Also, dental injuries can be associated with injuries to the maxillofacial region.[2] Therefore, make sure to evaluate for maxillofacial soft tissue injuries and fractures (see Chapter 5).

BRIEF ANATOMY REVIEW

Alveolar bone (sockets): The bony sockets that house the tooth root. Each tooth has its own socket.

Alveolar process: The stock of bone at the maxilla and mandible that houses the alveolar sockets, which hold the teeth.

Crown: The aspect of the tooth that is covered by the enamel.

Gingiva: Mucosa overlying the roots and surrounding the base of the tooth.

Lingual gland: Salivary gland located under the anterior aspect of the tongue.

Maxillary arch: The upper jaw. It is clinically divided into the left and right halves.

Mandibular arch: The lower jaw. It is clinically divided into the left and right halves. Therefore, the entire arch is divided into four quarters (left and right halves of the upper and lower jaw).

Parotid gland: Salivary gland located lateral to the second maxillary molars.

Periodontal ligament: The ligament that holds the teeth in the alveolar sockets. The ligament is comprised of many small fibers that line the cementum and connect the root to the socket walls.

Root: The aspect of the tooth that is covered by the cementum. The tip of the root is called the apex.

Submandibular gland: Salivary gland located under the floor of the mouth at the posterior half of the base of the mandible. Its duct extends to an opening at the frenulum of the tongue.

Teeth

Anterior Teeth

Incisors: The front teeth; there are two on each quarter.

Canines: The long sharp teeth located behind the incisors; there is one on each quarter.

Posterior Teeth

Premolars: Located behind the canines. The adult teeth have two premolars on each quarter.

Molars: The most posterior teeth, located behind the premolars. Deciduous teeth (baby teeth) have two molars, while the permanent teeth have three molars (third molar is a wisdom tooth) per quarter.

Tooth Tissues

Enamel: The hard visible tissue that forms the outermost layer of the tooth.

Cementum: The hard tissue that forms the outermost layer of the tooth, which is located under the gingival sulcus; it is not normally visible.

Dentin: The hard tissue that makes up the second layer of the tooth. Dentin makes up the bulk of the tooth.

Pulp: The soft tissue that makes up the innermost layer of the tooth. The pulp supplies the tooth with its arterial, venous, and nerve supply.

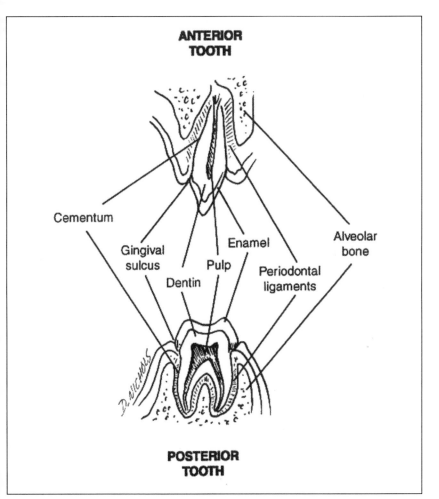

Figure 7-1. The anatomy of the tooth.

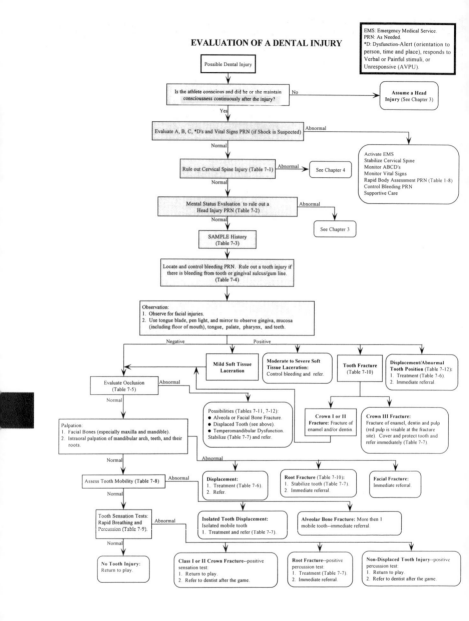

EVALUATION OF A DENTAL INJURY

EMS: Emergency Medical Service.
PRN: As Needed.
*D: Dysfunction-Alert (orientation to person, time and place), responds to Verbal or Painful stimuli, or Unresponsive (AVPU).

Possible Dental Injury

Is the athlete conscious and did he or she maintain consciousness continuously after the injury? — No → **Assume a Head Injury** (See Chapter 3)

Yes

Evaluate A, B, C, *D's and Vital Signs PRN (if Shock is Suspected) — Abnormal →

Normal

Rule out Cervical Spine Injury (Table 7-1) — Abnormal → See Chapter 4

Normal

Activate EMS
Stabilize Cervical Spine
Monitor ABCD's
Monitor Vital Signs
Rapid Body Assessment PRN (Table 1-8)
Control Bleeding PRN
Supportive Care

Mental Status Evaluation to rule out a Head Injury PRN (Table 7-2) — Abnormal →

Normal

See Chapter 3

SAMPLE History (Table 7-3)

Locate and control bleeding PRN. Rule out a tooth injury if there is bleeding from tooth or gingival sulcus/gum line. (Table 7-4)

Observation:
1. Observe for facial injuries.
2. Use tongue blade, pen light, and mirror to observe gingiva, mucosa (including floor of mouth), tongue, palate, pharynx, and teeth.

Negative   Positive

Mild Soft Tissue Laceration

Moderate to Severe Soft Tissue Laceration: Control bleeding and refer.

Tooth Fracture (Table 7-10)

Displacement/Abnormal Tooth Position (Table 7-12):
1. Treatment (Table 7-6).
2. Immediate referral.

Evaluate Occlusion (Table 7-5) — Abnormal →

Normal

Possibilities (Tables 7-11, 7-12):
● Alveola or Facial Bone Fracture.
● Displaced Tooth (see above).
● Temperomandibular Dysfunction.
Stabilize (Table 7-7) and refer.

Crown I or II Fracture: Fracture of enamel and/or dentin.

Crown III Fracture: Fracture of enamel, dentin and pulp (red pulp is visable at the fracture site). Cover and protect tooth and refer immediately (Table 7-7).

Palpation:
1. Facial Bones (especially maxilla and mandible).
2. Intraoral palpation of mandibular arch, teeth, and their roots.

Normal   Abnormal

Assess Tooth Mobility (Table 7-8) — Abnormal →

Normal

Displacement:
1. Treatment (Table 7-6).
2. Refer.

Root Fracture (Table 7-10):
1. Stabilize tooth (Table 7-7).
2. Immediate referral.

Facial Fracture: Immediate referral.

Tooth Sensation Tests: Rapid Breathing and Percussion (Table 7-9). — Abnormal →

Normal

Isolated Tooth Displacement: Isolated mobile tooth
1. Treatment and refer (Table 7-7).

Alveolar Bone Fracture: More then 1 mobile tooth--immediate referral.

No Tooth Injury: Return to play.

Class I or II Crown Fracture--positive sensation test:
1. Return to play.
2. Refer to dentist after the game.

Root Fracture--positive percussion test:
1. Treatment (Table 7-7).
2. Immediate referral.

Non-Displaced Tooth Injury--positive percussion test:
1. Return to play.
2. Refer to dentist after the game.

Table 7-1

Some Signs and Symptoms of a Significant Cervical Spine Injury[1,6]

- Involuntary loss of bowel and/or bladder control
- Cervical pain without movement
- Pain with palpation over the posterior or anterior cervical spine
- Rigid muscle spasms of the anterior and/or posterior neck muscles
- Deformity detected by palpation or the presence of a wryneck (abnormal neck position usually including flexion, rotation, and side bending)
- Decreased cervical spine mobility with pain
- Persistent burning, weakness, tingling, or numbness in any extremity

Table 7-2

Mental Status Evaluation[7,8]

AVPU (alert, responds to verbal or painful stimuli, or unresponsive) as indicated (Table 1-3).
Glasgow Coma Scale as needed and if time permits (Table 1-7).
Orientation to person, time, and place (Table 1-6).
Retrograde amnesia (loss of memory and events that occurred prior to the injury)—ask the athlete:
- What do you do on a certain play? (The clinician would need to ask about a specific play.)
- Do you know what play was run when the injury occurred?
- Do you know the score of the game?
- Do you know what team you played in the preceding game?

Post-traumatic amnesia (loss of memory and events that occur after the injury)—-ask the athlete:
- What do you first recall after the injury?
- Name four objects and have the athlete repeat them back immediately and 5 minutes later.

Ability to concentrate:
- Name the months of the year backward.
- Count backward from 100 in multiples of 3.

General impression after the evaluation:
- Facial expression: vacant stare or dazed look.
- Level of consciousness:
  - Alert: aware and responds appropriately and quickly to questions asked.
  - Lethargic: drowsy and falls asleep, but is easily aroused.
  - Stuporous: asleep most of the time and difficult to arouse; inappropriately responds to verbal stimuli.
  - Semicomatose: no response to verbal stimuli, but some reflexive response to pain.
  - Comatose: no response to verbal or painful stimuli; no motor activity.
- Speech patterns.
- Emotional state.
- Appropriate verbal and nonverbal responses to the above questions.

Table 7-3

SAMPLE History

Question	Indication
Symptoms	
Do you feel any sensitivity to hot, cold, or when breathing?	Class II or III crown fracture
Is there any sensitivity to closing the teeth or biting?	Root fracture; nondisplaced tooth injury
Do you feel that you can normally occlude your teeth (bring teeth together)?	Displaced tooth injury; alveolar process fracture
Allergies	
Do you have any known allergies?	This information may be helpful to a physician, dentist, or paramedic
Medications	
Are you currently taking any medications?	This information may be helpful to a physician, dentist, or paramedic
Past Medical History	
Do you have a root canal in one or more teeth?	A root canal will make the tests for sensation not valid when performed on the involved teeth
Are there any current or significant past history of dental problems?	The current injury could be an aggravation or progression of a previous injury
Are there any preexisting malocclusions or missing teeth?	It is important to know of any previous dental abnormalities prior to an evaluation
When was the last tetanus immunization you had? (Note: this question is only important in the presence of a wound)	Tetanus immunizations are effective for 10 years However, it may be wise for the athlete with a wound to have a "booster" shot if it has been longer then 5 years since the last tetanus shot
Last Meal Consumed	
When was the last time you ate or drank?	Knowledge of any recent meals may be helpful to a physician, dentist, or paramedic
Events Preceding the Injury	
Do you know how you hurt yourself?	This may help to differentiate between the possible type of dental injury the athlete may have

Table 7-4

Locate and Control Bleeding

1. Repeated blotting with gauze to locate the cause: soft tissue, tooth, or gingival sulcus/gum line (suspect a possible tooth injury if there is bleeding from the gingival sulcus).
2. Control bleeding by applying constant pressure with a gauze pad.
3. Debride the wound by flushing with saline, and assess the damage.

Table 7-5

Occlusion[9,10]

1. Ask about the presence of abnormal occlusion prior to the injury. This can be further clarified by seeing if the wear patterns of the teeth are occlusive with their counterparts.
2. Ask the athlete to close his or her jaws together.
   - The lips and cheeks should be retracted to allow proper viewing of the teeth.
   - Normally, the midline of the maxilla and mandible should line up.
   - Normally, the first maxillary incisors should slightly override the first mandibular incisors.
   - Ask the athlete if he or she perceives the occlusion to be normal.
   - If the athlete wears a custom mouth guard, check to see if it still fits properly. If the mouth guard does not fit the way it did prior to the injury, a malocclusion may be present.
   - Palpate over the masseter and temporalis muscles for symmetry of contraction (evaluates motor function of the trigeminal nerve/cranial nerve V).
   - If there is normal occlusion, a maxillary or mandible fracture can usually be ruled out.

Table 7-6

Initial Treatment of a Tooth Displacement[3,4]

Never forcefully realign or replant a displaced tooth.

Lateral Tooth Displacement (sideway dislocation of a tooth)

1. The examiner can try to manually guide the tooth back into place with digital pressure. The examiner should place his or her thumb and forefinger around the tooth and try to move the tooth as a unit.
2. Stabilize the tooth and immediately refer the athlete to a dentist.

Extrusion (partial avulsion of a tooth out of its socket)

1. The examiner can try to realign the tooth with digital pressure by gently pushing the tooth back into the socket.
2. The examiner can also have the athlete gently bite down on a piece of gauze in order to try to realign the displaced tooth.
3. Stabilize the tooth and immediately refer the athlete to a dentist.

Intrusion (displacement of a tooth into the alveolar socket)

1. Do not try to realign the tooth.
2. Stabilize the tooth and immediately refer the athlete to a dentist.

Avulsion (complete displacement a tooth)

Plan I. Try to replant the tooth if it has been avulsed for 30 minutes or less.

1. Hold the tooth by the crown only.
2. Gently rinse debris off of the root if needed. Use normal saline, or cold water if the above fluids are not available. If you cannot clean the tooth by rinsing, go to Plan II.
3. Do not scrub, chemically clean, or sterilize the root, as this will cause necrosis of the periodontal ligament.
4. Identify the front and back of the tooth.
5. If the tooth is clean, try to replant it back to its normal position using gentle force.
6. To check if the tooth has been realigned, use visual inspection and check for normal occlusion (see
   Chapter 5).
7. If the tooth cannot be realigned, it may be due to a hematoma in the alveolar socket. Try to rinse the socket with fluid (see step 2 above) in order to dislodge the clot.
8. Repeat step 5. If the tooth still will not go back with gentle pressure, then proceed to Plan II.
9. Refer the athlete immediately to a dentist.

Plan II. Follow the directions below if the tooth cannot be replanted or if it has been avulsed for more than 30 minutes.

1. Do not let the tooth dry out or wrap it in gauze or paper. This will cause necrosis of the periodontal ligament.
2. Do not place the tooth in tap water, as this will also cause periodontal necrosis.
3. Place the tooth in a medium during transportation. Use the media listed below. They are listed in importance from most to least desirable:
   a. Save-A-Tooth (3M Health Care)—keeps cells viable up to 12 hours.
   b. Balanced salt solution—keeps cells viable for 4 to 12 hours.
   c. Viaspan—keeps cells viable for 4 to 12 hours.
   d. Cold milk.
   e. Saliva—the tooth may be placed under the athlete's tongue, or place the tooth in a cup containing the athlete's saliva. When considering placing the tooth in the athlete's mouth, keep in mind the athlete's level of consciousness, mental status, and the presence of any intraoral bleeding.
   f. Normal saline.
4. Refer the athlete immediately to a dentist.

Table 7-7

Covering and/or Stabilizing Injured Teeth[4]

A tooth should be covered and/or stabilized in the event of a class III crown fracture, root fracture, fracture of the alveolar socket or process, or a displacement.

There are a few methods:

1. Cover the tooth with a piece of sterile gauze and then cover the gauze and tooth (along with surrounding teeth) with a piece of foil.
2. Have the athlete use his or her mouth guard. Make sure that the athlete does not forcefully bite the mouth guard.
3. Have the athlete gently bite down so that the upper and lower jaws occlude, preferably with piece of gauze between the upper and lower teeth.

Table 7-8

Assessing Tooth Mobility

Evaluate by placing the thumb and forefinger over the lingual (surface of the tooth that is adjacent to the tongue) and labial (surface of the tooth that is adjacent to the lips/cheeks) aspects of the tooth and attempt to move the tooth forward and backward.

1. First, check the mobility of an uninvolved tooth, far from the injury site, for a baseline of tooth movement.
2. Then, check the involved tooth. An isolated increase in tooth mobility is indicative of a root injury or tooth displacement.
3. Check the mobility of the adjacent teeth. Increased mobility is indicative of an alveolar process (bone) fracture.

Table 7-9

Tooth Sensation Tests[10]

1. Inhaled air test for thermal sensitivity: the athlete rapidly inhales air three times. This is painful in class I and II crown fractures.
2. Percussion test: gently tap the tooth with a hard object (end of a reflex hammer). This is painful in root fractures or nondisplaced tooth injuries.

Table 7-10
Tooth Injuries

Condition	Mechanism and General Information	Possible Signs/Symptoms
Crown fractures of enamel (class I fracture)	1. The tooth enamel is chipped, cracked, or fractured 2. The athlete can return to play but should follow up with a dentist after the game	1. Usually no tooth pain 2. May have pain from the sharp fracture edges rubbing against the soft tissues (tongue or lip)
Crown fractures of enamel and dentin (class II fracture)	1. A crown fracture that extends through the enamel and dentin 2. The athlete can return to play but should follow up with a dentist after the game	1. Tooth pain may be present 2. Thermal sensitivity
Crown fractures of the enamel, dentin, and pulp (class III fracture)	1. A crown fracture that extends through the enamel, dentin, and pulp 2. Exposure of the pulp can lead to an infection; cover the pulp and refer to a dentist as soon as possible	1. Mild to severe tooth pain 2. Thermal sensitivity 3. Red spot or drop of blood on the end of the tooth (at fracture site through the pulp)
Crown-root fracture	1. Horizontal or vertical fracture at or through the cementum-enamel junction 2. The pulp may be involved 3. Usually an unstable fracture; the periodontal ligament is holding the fragments together	1. Extremely painful 2. Very sensitive to palpation, even by the athlete's tongue or lips lightly touching the tooth
Root fracture	1. The fracture involves the cementum, dentin, and pulp 2. Often associated with alveolar bone fracture; check for mobility of adjacent teeth	1. Increased tooth mobility 2. Pain with percussion 3. Sensitivity to biting pressure 4. Palpable defect (can feel fracture site) over root during mobility testing

Table 7-11
Supporting Bone Injuries

Condition	Mechanism and General Information	Possible Signs/Symptoms
Fracture of alveola	1. Fracturing or shattering of alveolar socket or wall 2. Associated with a displaced tooth	See displaced tooth
Fracture of alveolar process	1. Fracture of alveolar bone (supporting bony structure of tooth socket) 2. Associated with mandible fractures and/or alveolar socket injuries	Increased mobility of two or more adjacent teeth
Fracture of jaw	See maxilla and mandible fractures in Chapter 5	See Chapter 5

Table 7-12

Periodontal and Soft Tissue Injuries

Condition	Mechanism and General Information	Possible Signs/Symptoms

Nondisplaced injuries	1. Trauma to periodontal ligaments; an injury to the pulp may also occur
	2. There are no obvious tooth deformities or abnormalities
	3. Problems may not be evident for weeks to months
	4. Two injury subtypes:
	  • Concussion: no loosening or displacement
	  • Subluxation: loosening, no displacement
		1. Sensitivity to percussion
		2. Sensitivity to palpation
		3. Hemorrhage at the gingival crevice
		If pulp necrosis occurs:
		1. Thermal and percussion sensitivity
		2. Tooth discoloration
		3. Swelling above the root apex

Displacement injuries	There are four types of displacement injuries:
	1. Extrusion: partial avulsion of the tooth out of its socket
	  • There is damage to the nerve, artery, vein, and pulp
	  • Can usually be reduced with manual digital pressure
	2. Lateral displacement: sideway dislocation of the tooth
	  • Associated with an alveolar socket fracture
	  • Can usually be reduced with manual digital pressure
	3. Intrusion: displacement of the tooth into the alveolar socket
	  • Associated with a fracture of the alveolar socket and pulp injury
	  • Do not attempt to reduce by pulling the tooth outward
	4. Avulsion: complete displacement of the tooth
	  • Primary concern is maintaining vitality of the periodontal ligament tissue that is remaining on the tooth
	  • Needs to be replanted within 30 minutes after injury or properly stored
		1. Pain
		2. Swelling
		3. Malocclusion (athlete complains that he or she is "biting wrong")
		4. Hemorrhage
		5. Increased tooth mobility
		6. Obvious displacement of crown and/or root (compared to normal or other teeth)

Soft tissue injuries	1. Laceration, abrasion, contusion, and/or puncture to the gingiva, oral mucosa, tongue palate, and/or pharynx 2. Profuse bleeding occurs due to the high vascularity of the oral soft tissues	1. Obvious profuse bleeding 2. Swelling 3. Pain 4. Subgingival or submucosal hematoma (secondary to a contusion) 5. Tongue trauma can lead to swelling, dysphagia (difficulty swallowing), drooling, dysgeusia (sensation of a bad taste in the mouth), and/or dysphonia (difficulty speaking)

References

1. Booher J, Thibodeau G. *Athletic Injury Assessment. 3rd ed.* St. Louis, Mo: Mosby; 1994:290-353.
2. Greenberg MS, Springer PS. Diagnosis and management of oral injuries. In: Torg JS, ed. *Athletic Injuries to the Head, Neck, and Face. 2nd ed.* St. Louis, Mo: Mosby-Year Book; 1991:635-649.
3. Wisniewski JF. Dental trauma. In: Andrews JR, Clancy WG, Whiteside JA, eds. *On-Field Evaluation and Treatment of Common Athletic Injuries.* St. Louis, Mo: Mosby; 1997:37-52.
4. Kurtz MD, Camp JH, Andreasen JO. Dental injuries. In: Scuderi G, McCann P, Bruno P, eds. *Sports Medicine: Principles of Primary Care.* St. Louis, Mo: Mosby; 1996:149-174.
5. Bakland LK, Boyne PJ. Trauma to the oral cavity. *Clin Sports Med.* 1989;8(1):25-41.
6. Torg JS, Ramsey-Emrhein JA. Cervical spine and brachial plexus injuries. *Phys Sportsmed.* 1997;25(7):61-88.
7. American Academy of Neurology. Practice parameter: the management of concussion in sports (summary statement). *Neurology.* 1997;48:581-585.
8. Price MB, DeVroom HL. A quick and easy guide to neurological assessment. *J Neurosurg Nurs.* 1985;17:313-320.
9. White MJ, Johnson PC, Heckler FR. Management of maxillofacial and neck soft-tissue injuries. *Clin Sports Med.* 1989;8:11-23.
10. Dreibelbeis MJ. Nonorthopedic problems. In: Sanders B, ed. *Sports Physical Therapy.* Norwalk, Conn: Appleton & Lange; 1990:273-287.

Bibliography

Castaldi CR. First aid for sports related dental injuries. *Phys Sportsmed.* 1987;15(9):81-89.
MacAfee KA. Immediate care of facial trauma. *Phys Sportsmed.* 1992;20:79-91.

CHAPTER 8

Thoracic Injuries

Thoracic injuries can be divided into thoracic wall injuries (anterior/chest, lateral, and posterior walls) and cardiopulmonary/intrathoracic injuries. Most injuries occur to the thoracic walls. Cardiopulmonary injuries are rare but can be fatal when they occur. Minor injuries to the thoracic walls, such as contusions and mild lacerations, sprains, and strains, can be managed at the sideline by the sports medicine clinician. However, serious thoracic wall injuries, such as severe lacerations, sprains, and strains, or fractures and/or subluxations/dislocations require a referral for a medical evaluation and treatment. All suspected cardiopulmonary injuries require a medical referral.

There are several landmarks to keep in mind during the evaluation. When examining the anterior chest, the manubriosternal junction (also known as the sternal angle or Louis' angle) can be palpated as a horizontal ridge on the superior sternum. The second rib articulates lateral to this line. The examiner can then count rib spaces from this reference point. The first six ribs attach directly to the sternum. It is difficult to palpate the intercostal spaces of the fourth to sixth ribs since the ribs are in close proximity. Anteriorly, the apex of the lungs extends above the clavicles. The anterioinferior aspect of the lungs is located under the sixth to eighth ribs.[1-3] During posterior examination, remember that the level of the thoracic vertebra correlates to the rib articulation (eg, the second rib attaches to the second thoracic vertebra). Posteriorly, the apex of the lungs extends to the level of the first rib, and the inferior aspect of the lungs is located under the 10th rib. The inferior angle of the scapula is usually lateral to the seventh thoracic vertebra spinous process while the athlete is standing with the arms at the sides.[1-3]

When evaluating for a potential cardiopulmonary injury in a child, remember that rib fracture in children is rare due to the large amount of rib elasticity. Therefore, always assume the possibility of other injuries (intra-abdominal or intrathoracic injuries) in the presence of a rib fracture in a child athlete.[4]

Hemoptysis (coughing or spitting blood or bloodstained sputum) is indicative of a serious cardiopulmonary injury. Hemoptysis can be difficult to differentiate from hematemesis (vomiting of blood), which indicates an injury to the intra-abdominal region. Possibly, a helpful clue to differentiate between the two conditions is to look for coagulation of blood at the gum line, which would indicate hematemesis.

This chapter occasionally refers to findings based on auscultation, percussion, and tactile fremitus.[3,5,6] These will briefly be discussed here, but it is beyond the scope of this book to explain indepth how to perform these evaluative techniques. Auscultation is listening to underlying tissues using a stethoscope. The clinician evaluates for the presence of normal sounds or adventitious (added) sounds. Adventitious sounds include:

1. Crackles: high-pitched and brief sounds that are indicative of abnormal lungs or airway.
2. Pleural rub: creaking sounds that are due to inflamed and roughened pleural surfaces rubbing against each other.

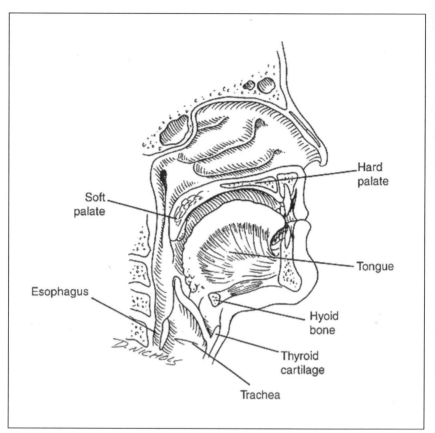

Figure 8-1. The anatomy of the upper airway and larynx (sagittal view).

3. Rhonchi: low-pitched snoring that is indicative of secretions in the airway.
4. Stridor: harsh, high-pitched, wheeze-like sound heard primarily during inspiration. Indicative of laryngeal edema or constriction.
5. Wheeze: a high-pitched hissing or musical sound that is heard primarily during inspiration and is indicative of a narrowed airway.

To perform percussion, percussive waves are created by tapping with the examiner's fingers to determine if the underlying tissues are filled with fluid, air, or a solid. Tactile fremitus is a palpable vibration of the chest wall created by the patient speaking, usually repeating the word "ninety-nine."[3,5,6] If the reader would like more information on these techniques, there are references listed at the end of the chapter.

BRIEF ANATOMY REVIEW

Hyoid bone: U-shaped bone located beneath the chin.

Larynx: the structure located between the pharynx and the trachea. The larynx contains the vocal cords and is supported by cartilage.

- Cricoid cartilage: a complete cartilaginous ring that is inferior to the thyroid cartilage.
- Thyroid cartilage: a V-shaped cartilage that houses the vocal cords. The anterior aspect is cartilage and the posterior aspect is muscle. It is larger in males (also known as the Adam's apple).

Lower airway: the region located from the inferior larynx to the alveoli of the lungs.

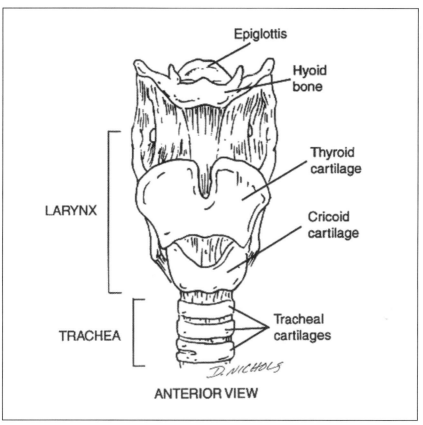

Figure 8-2. Anterior view of the larynx and trachea.

Lung parenchyma: the primary lobules of the lung. There are three lobes that constitute the right lung and two lobes that constitute the left lung.

Manubrium: the superior aspect of the sternum that articulates with the clavicle and the first and second ribs.

Mediastinum: the central region of the thoracic cavity that contains the heart, trachea, esophagus, great vessels, and several nerves.

Pericardium (or pericardial sac): the connective tissue that covers the heart, which consists of two basic layers.
- Fibrous pericardium: the outer layer, which is a strong fibrous connective tissue.
- Serous pericardium: a thin transparent membrane that is further divided into two layers.

Parietal pericardium: the layer of the serous pericardium that lines the fibrous pericardium.

Visceral pericardium (or epicardium): the layer of the serous pericardium that lines the heart muscle (myocardium).

Pericardial cavity: the potential space between the parietal and visceral pericardium.

Pharynx: the muscular tube that connects the oral and nasal cavities to the esophagus and trachea. Also known as the throat.

Pleura: the connective tissue that covers the lungs. There are two layers.
- Parietal pleura: connective tissue that lines the thoracic cavity.

- Visceral pleura: connective tissue that covers the lung. The cohesion between the two layers causes the lung to expand with the chest wall during inspiration.
- Pleural space: the potential space between the parietal and visceral pleura.

Trachea: the tube that connects the larynx to the bronchi. Its C-shaped cartilage rings support it.

Upper airway: the region from the mouth and nose to the larynx. This includes the nasal cavity, oral cavity, and the pharynx.

EVALUATION OF THORACIC INJURIES

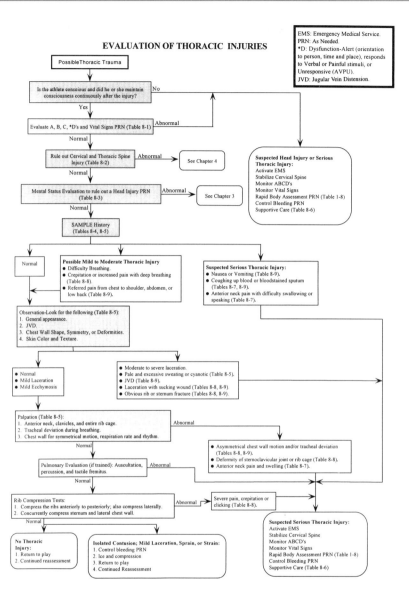

EMS: Emergency Medical Service.
PRN: As Needed.
*D: Dysfunction-Alert (orientation to person, time and place), responds to Verbal or Painful stimuli, or Unresponsive (AVPU).
JVD: Jugular Vein Distension.

Possible Thoracic Trauma

In the athlete conscious and did he or she maintain consciousness continuously after the injury? — No

Yes

Evaluate A, B, C, *D's and Vital Signs PRN (Table 8-1) — Abnormal

Normal

Rule out Cervical and Thoracic Spine Injury (Table 8-2) — Abnormal → See Chapter 4

Normal

Mental Status Evaluation to rule out a Head Injury PRN (Table 8-3) — Abnormal → See Chapter 3

Normal

SAMPLE History (Tables 8-4, 8-5)

Suspected Head Injury or Serious Thoracic Injury:
Activate EMS
Stabilize Cervical Spine
Monitor ABCD's
Monitor Vital Signs
Rapid Body Assessment PRN (Table 1-8)
Control Bleeding PRN
Supportive Care (Table 8-6)

Normal

Possible Mild to Moderate Thoracic Injury
● Difficulty Breathing.
● Crepitation or increased pain with deep breathing (Table 8-8).
● Referred pain from chest to shoulder, abdomen, or low back (Table 8-9).

Suspected Serious Thoracic Injury:
● Nausea or Vomiting (Table 8-9).
● Coughing up blood or bloodstained sputum (Tables 8-7, 8-9).
● Anterior neck pain with difficulty swallowing or speaking (Table 8-7).

Observation-Look for the following (Table 8-5):
1. General appearance.
2. JVD.
3. Chest Wall Shape, Symmetry, or Deformities.
4. Skin Color and Texture.

● Normal
● Mild Laceration
● Mild Ecchymosis

● Moderate to severe laceration.
● Pale and excessive sweating or cyanotic (Table 8-5).
● JVD (Table 8-9).
● Laceration with sucking wound (Tables 8-8, 8-9).
● Obvious rib or sternum fracture (Tables 8-8, 8-9).

Palpation (Table 8-5):
1. Anterior neck, clavicles, and entire rib cage.
2. Tracheal deviation during breathing.
3. Chest wall for symmetrical motion, respiration rate and rhythm. — Abnormal

Normal

● Asymmetrical chest wall motion and/or tracheal deviation (Tables 8-8, 8-9).
● Deformity of sternoclavicular joint or rib cage (Table 8-8).
● Anterior neck pain and swelling (Table 8-7).

Pulmonary Evaluation (if trained): Auscultation, percussion, and tactile fremitus. — Abnormal

Normal

Rib Compression Tests:
1. Compress the ribs anteriorly to posteriorly; also compress laterally.
2. Concurrently compress sternum and lateral chest wall. — Abnormal → Severe pain, crepitation or clicking (Table 8-8).

Normal

No Thoracic Injury:
1. Return to play
2. Continued reassessment

Isolated Contusion; Mild Laceration, Sprain, or Strain:
1. Control bleeding PRN
2. Ice and compression
3. Return to play
4. Continued Reassessment

Suspected Serious Thoracic Injury:
Activate EMS
Stabilize Cervical Spine
Monitor ABCD's
Monitor Vital Signs
Rapid Body Assessment PRN (Table 1-8)
Control Bleeding PRN
Supportive Care (Table 8-6)

Table 8-1

Vital Signs—Possible Abnormal Findings in the Presence of a Cardiopulmonary Injury*[1,7]

Sign	Abnormality	Interpretation
Breathing—rates	Tachypnea (rapid breathing) greater than 24 breaths/min Rapid and shallow Dyspnea (shortness of breath) less than eight breaths/min Possibly accompanied with deep, labored gasping and noisy	Shock, rib injuries, pneumothorax, hemothorax, cardiac contusion Partial airway obstruction; respiratory failure; moderate or severe pneumothorax or hemothorax; aorta rupture
Breathing—noises	Snoring Stridor/crowing Wheezing Gurgling Coughing	Partial airway obstruction Laryngeal obstruction 1. Lower airway obstruction 2. Asthma Fluid Pulmonary contusion/laceration
Pulse	Rapid Irregular	Pneumothorax; hemothorax; cardiac contusion Cardiac dysrythmia
Blood pressure[4,8]	Low blood pressure Decreasing systolic with possible increasing diastolic	Shock; hemothorax Tension pneumothorax; cardiac tamponade
Skin color and temperature	Pale and diaphoretic (profuse cool perspiration) Cyanosis of lips and nail beds	Early respiratory compromise; cardiac contusion; aorta rupture Late respiratory compromise

*See Table 1-2 for normal data

Table 8-2

Some Signs and Symptoms of a Significant Cervical Spine Injury[2,9]

- Involuntary loss of bowel and/or bladder control
- Cervical pain without movement
- Pain with palpation over the posterior or anterior cervical spine
- Rigid muscle spasms of the anterior and/or posterior neck muscles
- Deformity detected by palpation or the presence of a wryneck (abnormal neck position, usually including flexion, rotation, and side bending)
- Decreased cervical spine mobility with pain
- Persistent burning, weakness, tingling, or numbness in any extremity

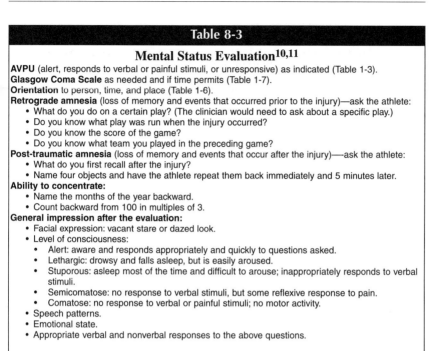

Table 8-3

Mental Status Evaluation[10,11]

AVPU (alert, responds to verbal or painful stimuli, or unresponsive) as indicated (Table 1-3).
Glasgow Coma Scale as needed and if time permits (Table 1-7).
Orientation to person, time, and place (Table 1-6).
Retrograde amnesia (loss of memory and events that occurred prior to the injury)—ask the athlete:
- What do you do on a certain play? (The clinician would need to ask about a specific play.)
- Do you know what play was run when the injury occurred?
- Do you know the score of the game?
- Do you know what team you played in the preceding game?

Post-traumatic amnesia (loss of memory and events that occur after the injury)—ask the athlete:
- What do you first recall after the injury?
- Name four objects and have the athlete repeat them back immediately and 5 minutes later.

Ability to concentrate:
- Name the months of the year backward.
- Count backward from 100 in multiples of 3.

General impression after the evaluation:
- Facial expression: vacant stare or dazed look.
- Level of consciousness:
  - Alert: aware and responds appropriately and quickly to questions asked.
  - Lethargic: drowsy and falls asleep, but is easily aroused.
  - Stuporous: asleep most of the time and difficult to arouse; inappropriately responds to verbal stimuli.
  - Semicomatose: no response to verbal stimuli, but some reflexive response to pain.
  - Comatose: no response to verbal or painful stimuli; no motor activity.
- Speech patterns.
- Emotional state.
- Appropriate verbal and nonverbal responses to the above questions.

Table 8-4

SAMPLE History

Question	Interpretation
Symptoms	
How severe is your pain and does deep breathing make the pain any worse?	Rib or sternum injury
Where is the pain located and does it radiate or refer somewhere else?	Pneumothorax
Is there the sensation of crepitation when you breathe?	Rib fracture
Do you have difficulty breathing?	Many possibilities
Have you been coughing or spitting up blood?	Pulmonary laceration or upper airway injury
Are you having any difficulty with swallowing or speaking?	Upper airway or tracheal injury
Are you having any nausea or have you been vomiting?	Possible cardiac contusion
Do you feel that you are getting better, worse, or staying the same?	Symptoms that stay the same or progressively worsen may indicate a serious thoracic injury
Allergies	
Do you have any known allergies?	This information may be helpful to a physician or paramedic
Medications	
Are you currently taking any medications?	This information may be helpful to a physician or paramedic
Past Medical History	
Do you have any current or past cardiopulmonary injuries or conditions?	The current injury could be an aggravation or progression of a previous injury
Last Meal Consumed	
When was the last time you ate or drank?	Knowledge of any recent meals may be helpful to a physician or paramedic
Events Preceding the Injury	
Do you know how you hurt yourself?	This may help to differentiate between the type of cardiopulmonary injury the athlete may have

Table 8-5

Some Serious Symptoms and Signs of a Thoracic Injury Requiring an Immediate Medical Referral

Symptom	Interpretation
Pleuratic pain (lateral chest pain) that is increased with twisting and coughing and decreased by sitting or leaning forward	Cardiac contusion
Anterior neck pain with airway compromise, vocal changes/dysphonia (difficulty speaking), and dysphagia (difficulty swallowing)	Anterior neck cartilage fracture (laryngeal fracture)
Respiratory distress or dyspnea (difficulty or labored breathing)	Many possibilities
Abnormal breathing sounds	Many possibilities
Hemoptysis (coughing or spitting blood or bloodstained sputum)	Many possibilities
Subcutaneous emphysema (a palpable subcutaneous crackling sensation due to air collection in soft tissues)	Several possibilities
Tracheal deviation	Fractured trachea, simple or tension pneumothorax, hemothorax, traumatic aorta rupture
Palpable defects and/or crepitus along the rib cage (ribs, sternum, mandubrium, clavicle)	Fracture
Asymmetrical breath sounds or chest wall movements with breathing	Fracture, pneumothorax
Rib cage compression tests positive for rib pain	Fracture
Skin color changes (pale or cyanosis)	Respiratory compromise
Uncontrolled tachypnea (rapid breathing)	Pneumothorax, hemothorax, cardiac contusion
Uncontrolled tachycardia (rapid heart rate)	Cardiac contusion
Jugular vein distention (JVD): below 45 degrees of body elevation (supine), mild JVD normally occurs; in an upright position, no JVD should be present	Tension pneumothorax, cardiac tamponade
Nausea and vomiting	Cardiac contusion
Hypotension	Several possibilities
Pale, sweaty, thirsty, rapid and tready pulse, hypotension, and delayed capillary refill	Hypovolemic shock

Make an immediate medical referral whenever in doubt regarding the seriousness of the injury

Table 8-6

Supportive Care for the Occurrence of a Serious Thoracic Injury[2]

1. Activate the EMS.
2. Act calm and reassuring so that the athlete can relax and breathe easier.
3. Keep airway clear of any foreign bodies, blood, or vomitus.
4. Find the most comfortable position for the athlete to breathe.
5. Be prepared to provide CPR if needed.
6. Do not give food, fluids, or pain medications to the athlete.

Table 8-7

Traumatic Anterior Neck Injuries

Condition	Mechanism and General Information	Possible Signs/Symptoms
Contusion with soft tissue injury	1. Caused by blunt neck trauma 2. Can cause a hematoma and/or edema can develop, which can enlarge and cause an airway obstruction 3. Can also cause an isolated vocal cord injury, mucosal tear, pharynx rupture, or esophagus rupture 4. Vocal cord changes can be delayed due to accumulation of edema over time	1. Anterior neck pain 2. Palpable hematoma in anterior neck 3. Vocal changes 4. Respiratory distress 5. Dysphagia (difficulty swallowing)
Fracture of the hyoid, thyroid cartilage, cricoid cartilage, and/or trachea	1. Caused by a forceful blow to the anterior neck 2. Usually will cause hemorrhage and edema with possible laryngeal nerve compression, laryngospasm, and/or subcutaneous emphysema (a palpable subcutaneous crackling sensation due to air collection in the soft tissues)	Three major signs: 1. Airway compromise 2. Vocal changes from hoarseness to aphonia (inability to speak) 3. Difficulty swallowing from dysphagia to complete inability to swallow Others: 1. Coughing 2. Stridor (wheeze), especially on inspiration 3. Loss of neck contour with observation and palpation 4. Hemoptysis (coughing or spitting of blood or bloodstained sputum) 5. Neck swelling 6. Subcutaneous emphysema 7. Ipsilateral tracheal deviation 8. Anxiety due to breathing difficulties

Table 8-8

Traumatic Thoracic Wall Injuries

Condition	Mechanism and General Information	Possible Signs/Symptoms
Breast trauma	Caused by a contusion or, in females, stretching of Cooper's suspensory ligaments (usually from running)	1. Localized pain and swelling.
Costovertebal joint sprain	Usually caused by the forceful movement of flexion, rotation, and side bending	1. Sharp posterior thoracic pain and/or a "catching" sensation with movement or possibly with deep breathing 2. Pain with passive vertebral movement 3. Pain may be felt over the anterior chest as well as posteriorly
Pectoralis major tear	1. Caused by a forceful muscle contraction or a blow to the shoulder with the shoulder in abduction and external rotation 2. Usually tears at the lateral musculotendon junction	1. Sharp sudden pain 2. Hearing a snap or pop at the time of injury 3. Pain and weakness 4. Ecchymosis and swelling 5. Palatable defect 6. Bulge of muscle with contraction
Effort thrombosis (of the subclavian or axillary vein)	1. Caused by a single traumatic event to the clavicular/shoulder area or an overuse injury of repetitive overhead movements	1. Pain 2. Swelling of ipsilateral arm 3. Possible numbness
Sternoclavicular joint dislocation	1. Caused by a force that compresses and protracts the shoulder or by a posteriorly directed force to the medial clavicle 2. The clavicle usually dislocates anteriorly 3. A posterior dislocation is potentially more dangerous and can cause injury to the great vessels, trachea, esophagus, lung laceration, and pneumothorax	For a posterior dislocation: 1. Painful and palpable defect 2. Swelling 3. Decreased function of the upper extremity 4. Dyspnea (difficult or labored breathing) 5. Stridor (wheeze) with auscultation 6. Dysphonia (difficulty speaking) 7. Choking 8. Coughing
Sternum fracture	1. Caused by a direct blow to the sternum with a high force or a trunk hyperflexion injury 2. The manubrium is usually held in place while the sternum is driven posteriorly; the sternum can reduce or remain displaced 3. There may be a secondary myocardial contusion, aorta disruption, flail chest, pneumothorax, or hemothorax	1. Immediate loss of breath 2. Localized sternal tenderness and/or defect 3. Swelling 4. Pain with normal respirations 5. Increased pain with inspirations 6. If the manubrium is displaced posteriorly, there will be an airway obstruction
Rib contusion	Caused by a direct blow with secondary bruising of the intercostal muscles	1. Pain, primarily due to muscle spasm 2. Difficulty breathing 3. Reproducible sharp pain with inspiration and expiration 4. Localized tenderness 5. Swelling 6. No crepitus or asymmetrical breath sounds

Table 8-8, continued

Condition	Mechanism and General Information	Possible Signs/Symptoms
Rib fractures	1. Caused by a direct blow or compression of the ribs 2. Ribs four through nine are the most commonly fractured ribs, usually fracturing at the mid axillary line 3. Can cause a secondary pneumothorax, hemothorax, lung laceration, or penetration of the pericardium. Additionally, a lower rib fracture can cause an injury to the liver, spleen, or kidney. 4. A flail chest can occur if more than three successive ribs are fractured at two or more sites	1. Pain with secondary decreased ventilation 2. Shallow rapid breathing 3. Swelling secondary to a hematoma of the intercostal vessels 4. Increased pain with deep breathing, coughing, or sneezing 5. Palpable defect and crepitation 6. Pain with the rib compression test 7. Athlete grabbing chest to decrease movement 8. Dyspnea and cyanosis 9. Asymmetrical breath sounds if the fracture is complicated 10. In a flail chest, the unstable ribs move in the opposite direction of the chest wall (paradoxical movement)
First rib fracture	1. Causes include direct trauma, a violent muscle contraction, a fall on an outstretched hand, or with a hyperabduction force at the glenohumoral joint. 2. Secondarily, there can be a laceration of the lung apex, pleurisy, aortic arch or subclavian injury, or a brachial plexus syndrome	1. Sensation of a snap in the shoulder during the injury 2. Acute pain, which may be located in the infrascapular region 3. Increased pain with shoulder movement and possibly neck movement 4. Shoulder weakness and decreased movement 5. Swelling
Costochondral sprain and/or dislocation	1. Causes include a direct blow to the rib-sternum junction, rib cage compression, or the ipsilateral arm pulled/distracted outward 2. With a dislocation, there is separation of the anterior rib cartilage from the sternum or rib body 3. With a sprain, there is inflammation at the anterior rib-cartilage junction	1. Sharp pain localized to the costochondral junction 2. When the dislocated cartilage reduces, there is a click with a decrease in pain 3. Increased pain with coughing and sneezing 4. Palpable tenderness with a defect if the rib is displaced 5. Pain and a possible click (if dislocated) with a medially directed force to the rib during a concurrent posteriorly directed force on the sternum

Table 8-9

Traumatic Intrathoracic Injuries

Condition	Mechanism and General Information	Possible Signs/Symptoms
Diaphragmatic injuries	1. Diaphragmatic paralysis due to a root avulsion of the phrenic nerve; this can occur during a forceful cervical flexion and rotation injury (similar to the mechanism of injury involving the brachial plexus)	Diaphragmatic paralysis: 1. Pain radiating to the upper trapezius 2. Dyspnea with exertion 3. Dullness to percussion 4. Decreased breath sounds with auscultation
	2. Celiac (solar) plexus syndrome occurs due to a blow to the middle to upper abdomen that causes transient paralysis of the diaphragm	Celiac plexus syndrome: 1. Shortness of breath 2. Coughing 3. Hemoptysis 4. Respiratory difficulty/shortness of breath 5. Auscultation may reveal decreased breath sounds and/or rales (fine crackles)
Pulmonary contusion/laceration	1. Causes include a deceleration injury, blunt trauma, or displaced rib fracture 2. Most cases are mild and asymptomatic 3. Hypoxia can develop 2 to 4 hours after the injury due to development of interstitial edema 4. A lung laceration can secondarily cause hemorrhage, infection, pneumothorax, or hemothorax	
Pneumothorax	1. A unidirectional air leak from a lung into the pleural space that causes a partial or complete collapse of the lung 2. Causes: • Spontaneous: spontaneous rupture of a lung bleb; may be caused by coughing or exertion (may occur after exercise) • Compression: compressive forces that tear the lung • Laceration: displaced rib lacerates the lung	Simple pneumothorax: 1. Chest pain, which may radiate to the neck, abdomen, or low back 2. Tachypnea (rapid breathing) 3. Dyspnea 4. Shortness of breath 5. Decreased tactile fremitus 6. Decreased breath sounds with auscultation 7. Hyper-resonance with percussion 8. Ipsilateral tracheal deviation 9. Mild cases are usually asymptomatic
	3. Tension pneumothorax: increasing pleural pressure causes the lung to collapse and presses against the heart and contralateral lung, decreasing their function	Tension pneumothorax: 1. Same as 1 through 7 above 2. Tachycardia (rapid heart rate) 3. JVD 4. Hypotension 5. Contralateral tracheal shift 6. Referred pain to contralateral shoulder

Table 8-9, continued

Condition	Mechanism and General Information	Possible Signs/Symptoms
Open pneumothorax (sucking chest wound)	1. External opening of the chest wall due to a penetrating injury or a complicated rib fracture 2. Air enters the pleural space during inspiration	1. Obvious deformity of the outer chest wall 2. Sucking sound with inspiration
Hemothorax	1. Similar to a pneumothorax, but blood enters the pleural space instead of air 2. Caused by injured vessels in the chest wall, chest cavity, or fractured rib 3. Can occur in conjunction with a pneumothorax, called a hemo-pneumothorax	1. Same as for a pneumothorax 2. May have shock due to blood loss 3. May have hemoptysis
Cardiac contusion	1. A heart bruise that can be caused by blunt chest trauma, deceleration (contracoup injury), or, rarely, a sudden increase in intra-thoracic pressure 2. Rarely, it can cause a myocardial infarction due to the development of a thrombosis or coronary artery spasm	1. Chest pain 2. Pleuritic pain, which may be increased by twisting or coughing and decreased by sitting or leaning forward 3. Tachycardia 4. Tachypnea 5. Diaphoretic (profuse perspiration) 6. Nausea and vomiting 7. Muffled heart sounds on auscultation
Commotio cordis	1. Caused by a direct blow to the chest wall, which disrupts cardiac electrical activity, leading to cardiac arrhythmias 2. Low survival rate	1. Sudden collapse after a blow to the chest 2. Unresponsive
Cardiac tamponade	A blunt injury to the chest or upper abdomen that causes an accu-mulation of fluid between the pericardium and the heart	1. Hypotension 2. JVD 3. Muffled heart sounds on auscultation
Traumatic aorta rupture	1. High speed deceleration injury that causes a rupture, usually distal to the subclavian artery 2. The injury can also occur due to a laceration from a first or second rib fracture 3. Most severe ruptures are fatal 4. There can be a small rupture with no symptoms or a delayed onset of symptoms	1. Sudden collapse and unresponsive may be the only signs 2. Right tracheal deviation 3. Unexplained hypotension If the rupture is small: 1. Chest pain 2. Dyspnea 3. Diaphoretic 4. Anuria (cessation of urine production by the kidneys) 5. Hypertension of one or both upper extremities

References

1. Bledsoe B, Porter R, Shade B. *Brady Paramedic Emergency Care. 3rd ed.* Upper Saddle River, NJ: Brady Prentice Hall; 1997:205-283, 469-497.
2. Booher J, Thibodeau G. *Athletic Injury Assessment. 3rd ed.* St. Louis, Mo: Mosby; 1994:316-395.
3. Bates B, Bickley LS, Hoekelman RA. *A Guide to Physical Examination and History Taking. 6th ed.* Philadelphia, Pa: JB Lippincott Co; 1991:229-258.
4. Cogbill TH, Landercasper J. Injury to the chest wall. In: Feliciano DV, Moore EE, Mattox KL, eds. *Trauma. 3rd ed.* Stamford, Conn: Appelton & Lange; 1996:487-523.
5. Arnall D, Ryan M. Screening for pulmonary system disease. In: Boissonnault WG, ed. *Examination in Physical Therapy Practice. 2nd ed.* New York, NY: Churchill Livingstone; 1995:69-100.
6. *Assessment Review Series: Respiratory System.* Videotape. Springhouse Corp; 1992.
7. Erickson SM, Rich BE. Pulmonary and chest wall emergencies. *Phys Sportsmed.* 1995;23(11):95-104.
8. Athletic Training Emergency Care. *Course Notebook.* Wichita, Ks. April 1997 (c/o DCH Outpatient Services, 809 University Boulevard East, Tuscaloosa, AL 35401).
9. Torg JS, Ramsey-Emrhein JA. Cervical spine and brachial plexus injuries. *Phys Sportsmed.* 1997;25(7):61-88.
10. American Academy of Neurology. Practice parameter: the management of concussion in sports (summary statement). *Neurology.* 1997;48:581-585.
11. Price MB, DeVroom HL. A quick and easy guide to neurological assessment. *J Neurosurg Nurs.* 1985;17:313-320.

Bibliography

Amaral JF. Thoracoabdominal injuries in the athlete. *Clin Sports Med.* 1997;16:739-753.

Bragg LE. Athletic injuries of the thorax and abdomen. In: Mellion M, Walsh W, Shelton G, eds. *The Team Physician's Handbook.* Philadelphia, Pa: Hanley & Belfus; 1990:365-373.

Browne RJ. Chest injuries. In: Andrews JR, Clancy WG, Whiteside JA, eds. *On-Field Evaluation and Treatment of Common Athletic Injuries.* St. Louis, Mo: Mosby; 1997:53-62.

Espinosa R, Badui E, Castano R, Madrid R. Acute posterioinferior wall myocardial infarction secondary to football chest trauma. *Chest.* 1985;88:926-929.

Fabian RL. Sports injury to the larynx and trachea. *Phys Sportsmed.* 1989;17(2):111-118.

Handler SD. Diagnosis and management of maxillofacial injuries. In: Torg JS, ed. *Athletic Injuries to the Head, Neck, and Face. 2nd ed.* St. Louis, Mo: Mosby-Year Book; 1991:611-634.

Johnson MB, Haines M, Barry B. Recognizing pneumothorax—a case study. *Athletic Therapy Today.* 1996;1(6):42-46.

Lowery DW. Soft tissue trauma of the head and neck. *Phys Sportsmed.* 1991;19(10):21-24.

Marino N, Bruno P. Cardiopulmonary conditions. In: Scuderi G, McCann P, Bruno P, eds. *Sports Medicine: Principles of Primary Care.* St. Louis, Mo: Mosby; 1996:18-34.

Richardson JD, Miller FB. Injury to the lung and pleura. In: Feliciano DV, Moore EE, Mattox KL, eds. *Trauma. 3rd ed.* Stamford, Conn: Appelton & Lange; 1996:387-407.

Storey MD, Schatz CF, Brown KW. Anterior neck trauma. *Phys Sportsmed.* 1989;17(9):85-96.

Volk CP, McFarland EG, Horsmon G. Pneumothorax: on-field recognition. *Phys Sportsmed.* 1995;23(10):43-46.

Wagner GS, Sidhu GS, Radcliffe WB. Pulmonary contusion in contact sports. *Phys Sportsmed.* 1992;20(2):126-136.

Yates MT, Aldrete V. Blunt trauma causing aortic rupture. *Phys Sportsmed.* 1991;19(11):96-107.

CHAPTER 9

Abdominal Injuries

As with thoracic injuries, abdominal injuries can be divided into abdominal wall injuries and intra-abdominal injuries. Making an assessment after performing an abdominal exam can be challenging. It is difficult to assess if an injury has occurred to a specific intra-abdominal organ. Instead of trying to make a specific assessment, this chapter's algorithm helps the clinician decide if there is an isolated abdominal wall injury or the possibility of a more serious intra-abdominal injury (either of acute onset or slowly developing). An isolated mild to moderate abdominal wall injury can be managed at the sideline by the sports medicine clinician. However, a severe abdominal wall injury or any suspicion of an intra-abdominal injury would require that the athlete be immediately referred for medical evaluation and treatment. A combination of the two injury types could occur, which would obviously require a medical referral.[1] When in doubt about whether an intra-abdominal injury has occurred, refer the athlete for a medical evaluation. Waiting to see if more signs develop may be harmful since an initially mild injury can rapidly progress to a life-threatening injury.

The most common mechanism of abdominal injury is blunt trauma to the abdomen. Other mechanisms of injury include deceleration (contracoup injuries), penetrating injuries, and injuries due to a rapid and severe increase in intra-abdominal pressure. The most commonly injured abdominal organs are the spleen, kidneys, and liver.[2] Injuries to solid organs (liver, spleen, pancreas, kidneys, adrenal, and ovaries) are manifested by hemorrhage, while injury to hollow organs (stomach, intestines, gall bladder, urinary bladder, and uterus) are manifested by chemical or bacterial peritoneal irritation secondary to leakage by rupture.[3] Hollow organs are more susceptible to injury if they are full of food, waste, or fluids.[4] It is also important to note that during maximum expiration, the diaphragm can rise superiorly to the fourth intercostal space. Thus, lower thoracic trauma during full expiration can injure the liver, spleen, stomach, gallbladder, and transverse colon.[5]

It can be very difficult to evaluate an intra-abdominal injury for several reasons.[5] First, due the anatomical proximity and overlapping of organs, it is difficult to palpate for a specific intra-abdominal structure. Second, the abdominal organs are mostly insensitive to pain due to the lack of pain fibers. Isolated injuries to the abdominal organ may not develop much pain unless the organ capsule is involved, which is innervated with pain fibers. The exception is the liver, which is highly innervated with pain fibers.[4] Third, peritoneal irritation by the presence of blood is usually the initial sign of an intra-abdominal injury. The pain usually starts at the site of injury. As the peritoneum is further irritated, the pain radiates to include the entire abdomen. However, the abdominal cavity is a large space for blood to accumulate and the peritoneum is not very sensitive to blood. Thus, it can take hours to days for this pain to occur.[6] Fourth, auscultation for bowel sounds may not be a reliable tool for assessing visceral damage. Although diminished bowel sounds are a sign of intra-abdominal injury, they can be caused by many factors not associated with visceral injury. This includes dehydration, electrolyte disorders, spinous process fractures, or the sympathetic response to exercise.[7]

Intra-abdominal injuries are usually subtle in presentation and therefore have the potential to be unrecognized and/or poorly treated.[6] A serious injury can have no initial signs or symptoms and can take hours or days to manifest. Meanwhile, an abdominal wall injury can initially have pain and disability that a more serious injury would not have.[8] Up to 40% of athletes with serious abdominal injuries initially have a normal physical examination.[5] Therefore, it should be assumed that an athlete who receives a blow to the abdominal region has a severe injury until proven otherwise. Also, all abdominal complaints should be taken seriously.[2,9] Most intra-abdominal injuries require serial examinations performed by the same examiner to find subtle changes, which can be indicative of a serious injury.[5]

However, some intra-abdominal injuries have an acute presentation. A severe intra-abdominal injury can cause acute excessive bleeding, and the athlete can quickly develop hypovolemic shock.[6] Also, traumatic injuries to the stomach, gall bladder, pancreas, small intestine, and colon can cause severe pain if there is chemical and bacterial leakage, which irritates the peritoneum.[6] Therefore, signs of peritoneal irritation or shock are indicative of a serious intra-abdominal injury.

The abdomen and genital regions are close in proximity and have several interrelationships. For example, in females many reproductive organs are located in the peritoneal cavity. In males, the vas deferens travels between the external genitalia and the peritoneal cavity. Thus, the evaluation of injuries to these separate regions were combined in this chapter. It is best to have a physician perform a genital exam. However, a physician may not be present when a genital evaluation is needed. If the clinician feels uncomfortable performing a screening evaluation of the genital region, the exam should be referred to another individual. For media-legal reasons, a third party should be present when performing a genital evaluation.

BRIEF ANATOMY REVIEW

Abdominal-pelvic cavity (peritoneal cavity): the cavity that is bound superiorly by the diaphragm and inferiorly by the pelvic floor. It contains all of the intra-abdominal organs. All of these structures are covered with peritoneum.

Epididymis: the duct located posterior to the testes that is a storage and maturation site for sperm.

Glands: the end of the penis that is covered with a mucous membrane.

Large intestine: the digestive tube that starts at the small intestine and ends at the rectum. It is comprised of the ascending colon, transverse colon, descending colon, sigmoid colon, and the rectum.

Mesentery: double layer of peritoneum that attaches portions of the intestine to the posterior body wall and supplies it with blood vessels and nerves.

Omentum: double layer of peritoneum that hangs in front of the abdominal organs and acts as a protective layer against trauma and temperature changes.

Penis: the male organ used for reproduction and urination.

Peritoneum: the tissue that covers the interior walls and organs of the abdominal cavity. It is very sensitive and can easily be irritated by the presence of bodily fluids.

Retroperitoneal cavity: cavity in the posterior abdomen that contains the kidneys, aorta, inferior vena cava, and portions of the duodenum and pancreas. These organs are not covered with peritoneum.

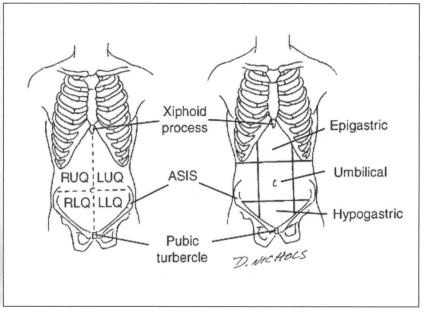

Figure 9-1. Quadrants and regions of the abdomen.

Small intestine: the digestive tube that extends from the stomach to the large intestine. It is comprised of three parts: the duodenum, jejunum, and ileum.

Spermatic cord: the cord, formed by layers of the abdominal wall, that contains the structures that go to and from the testis (vas deferens, arteries, veins, nerves, and lymph vessels).

Testes: the male gonad where the sperm is produced.

Urethra: the tube that carries urine from the bladder to the exterior of the body.

Urinary meatus: the opening of the urethra to the exterior of the body.

Vas deferens: the duct that carries sperm from the epididymis to the ejaculatory duct.

Vulva: the collective region of the external female genital organs.

For examination purposes, the abdomen is divided into four quadrants and two regions. The vertical and horizontal lines that make the quadrants intersect at the umbilicus:[14,15]

Right upper quadrant: liver, right kidney, gall bladder, duodenum, distal portion of the ascending colon, proximal part of the transverse colon, and part of the pancreas.

Left upper quadrant: left kidney, spleen, distal portion of the transverse colon, and proximal portion of the descending colon.

Right lower quadrant: appendix, cecum, right ovary, and proximal portion of the ascending colon.

Left lower quadrant: distal portion of the descending colon, sigmoid colon, and left ovary.

Epigastric region (located inferior to the xiphiod process): stomach and pancreas.

Suprapubic region (located superior to pubic bones): uterus and bladder.

Additionally, the organs in the abdomen can be divided into two types.[14] The solid organs include the liver, spleen, pancreas, kidneys, adrenal, and ovaries. The hollow organs include the stomach, intestines, gall bladder, urinary bladder, and uterus.

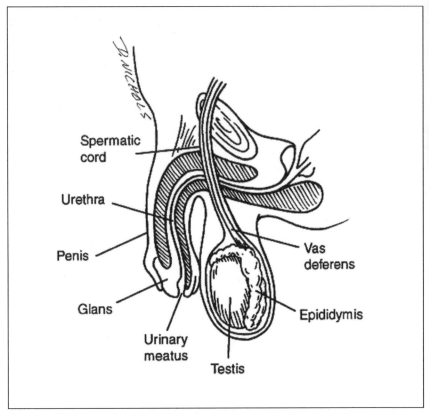

Figure 9-2. The anatomy of the male genital region.

EVALUATION OF AN ABDOMINAL INJURY

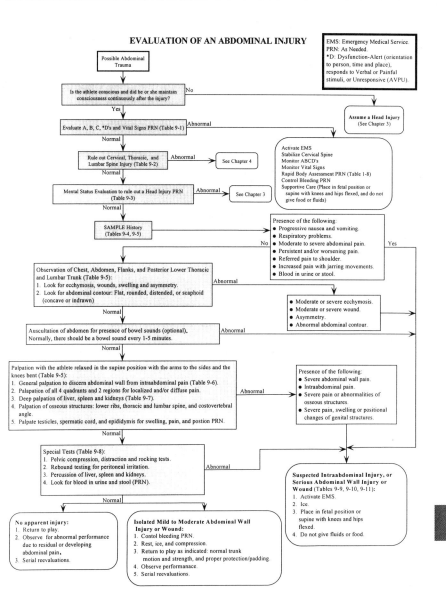

EMS: Emergency Medical Service.
PRN: As Needed.
*D: Dysfunction-Alert (orientation to person, time and place), responds to Verbal or Painful stimuli, or Unresponsive (AVPU).

Possible Abdominal Trauma

Is the athlete conscious and did he or she maintain consciousness continuously after the injury? — No → **Assume a Head Injury** (See Chapter 3)

Yes

Evaluate A, B, C, *D's and Vital Signs PRN (Table 9-1) — Abnormal →

Normal

Rule out Cervical, Thoracic, and Lumbar Spine Injury (Table 9-2) — Abnormal → See Chapter 4

Normal

Mental Status Evaluation to rule out a Head Injury PRN (Table 9-3) — Abnormal → See Chapter 3

Activate EMS
Stabilize Cervical Spine
Monitor ABCD's
Monitor Vital Signs
Rapid Body Assessment PRN (Table 1-8)
Control Bleeding PRN
Supportive Care (Place in fetal position or supine with knees and hips flexed, and do not give food or fluids)

Normal

SAMPLE History (Tables 9-4, 9-5)

Presence of the following:
● Progressive nausea and vomiting.
● Respiratory problems.
● Moderate to severe abdominal pain.
● Persistent and/or worsening pain.
● Referred pain to shoulder.
● Increased pain with jarring movements.
● Blood in urine or stool.

No / Yes

Observation of Chest, Abdomen, Flanks, and Posterior Lower Thoracic and Lumbar Trunk (Table 9-5):
1. Look for ecchymosis, wounds, swelling and asymmetry.
2. Look for abdominal contour: Flat, rounded, distended, or scaphoid (concave or indrawn) — Abnormal →

● Moderate or severe ecchymosis.
● Moderate or severe wound.
● Asymmetry.
● Abnormal abdominal contour.

Normal

Auscultation of abdomen for presence of bowel sounds (optional). Normally, there should be a bowel sound every 1-5 minutes. — Abnormal →

Normal

Palpation with the athlete relaxed in the supine position with the arms to the sides and the knees bent (Table 9-5):
1. General palpation to discern abdominal wall from intraabdominal pain (Table 9-6).
2. Palapation of all 4 quadrants and 2 regions for localized and/or diffuse pain.
3. Deep palpation of liver, spleen and kidneys (Table 9-7).
4. Palpation of osseous structures: lower ribs, thoracic and lumbar spine, and costovertebral angle.
5. Palpate testicles, spermatic cord, and epididymis for swelling, pain, and postion PRN. — Abnormal →

Presence of the following:
● Severe abdominal wall pain.
● Intraabdominal pain.
● Severe pain or abnormalities of osseous structures.
● Severe pain, swelling or positional changes of genital structures.

Normal

Special Tests (Table 9-8):
1. Pelvic compression, distraction and rocking tests.
2. Rebound testing for peritoneal irritation.
3. Percussion of liver, spleen and kidneys.
4. Look for blood in urine and stool (PRN). — Abnormal →

Normal

No apparent injury:
1. Return to play.
2. Observe for abnormal performance due to residual or developing abdominal pain.
3. Serial reevaluations.

Isolated Mild to Moderate Abdominal Wall Injury or Wound:
1. Contol bleeding PRN.
2. Rest, ice, and compression.
3. Return to play as indicated: normal trunk motion and strength, and proper protection/padding.
4. Observe performace.
5. Serial reevaluations.

Suspected Intraabdominal Injury, or Serious Abdominal Wall Injury or Wound (Tables 9-9, 9-10, 9-11):
1. Activate EMS.
2. Ice.
3. Place in fetal position or supine with knees and hips flexed.
4. Do not give fluids or food.

Table 9-1

Vital Signs—Possible Abnormal Findings in an Abdominal Injury[6]

A severe abdominal injury can cause excessive bleeding, and an athlete can quickly develop hypovolemic shock, which has some of the following signs and symptoms.

- Pale
- Sweaty
- Thirsty
- Rapid and weak pulse
- Hypotension
- Delayed capillary refill

Table 9-2

Some Signs and Symptoms of a Significant Spine Injury[4,10]

- Involuntary loss of bowel and/or bladder control
- Spine pain without movement
- Pain with palpation over the posterior or anterior cervical spine
- Pain with palpation over the thoracic or lumbar spine
- Rigid muscle spasms of the anterior and/or posterior neck muscles
- Deformity detected by palpation or the presence of a wryneck (abnormal neck position usually including flexion, rotation, and side bending)
- Decreased spine mobility with pain
- Persistent burning, weakness, tingling, or numbness in any extremity
- Thoracic spine pain with deep breathing

Table 9-3

Mental Status Evaluation[11,12]

AVPU (alert, responds to verbal or painful stimuli, or unresponsive) as indicated (Table 1-3).
Glasgow Coma Scale as needed and if time permits (Table 1-7).
Orientation to person, time, and place (Table 1-6).
Retrograde amnesia (loss of memory and events that occurred prior to the injury)—ask the athlete:
- What do you do on a certain play? (The clinician would need to ask about a specific play.)
- Do you know what play was run when the injury occurred?
- Do you know the score of the game?
- Do you know what team you played in the preceding game?

Post-traumatic amnesia (loss of memory and events that occur after the injury)—ask the athlete:
- What do you first recall after the injury?
- Name four objects and have the athlete repeat them back immediately and 5 minutes later.

Ability to concentrate:
- Name the months of the year backward.
- Count backward from 100 in multiples of 3.

General impression after the evaluation:
- Facial expression: vacant stare or dazed look.
- Level of consciousness:
  - Alert: aware and responds appropriately and quickly to questions asked.
  - Lethargic: drowsy and falls asleep, but is easily aroused.
  - Stuporous: asleep most of the time and difficult to arouse; inappropriately responds to verbal stimuli.
  - Semicomatose: no response to verbal stimuli, but some reflexive response to pain.
  - Comatose: no response to verbal or painful stimuli; no motor activity.
- Speech patterns.
- Emotional state.
- Appropriate verbal and nonverbal responses to the above questions.

Table 9-4

SAMPLE History

Question	Interpretation
Symptoms	
Did the pain begin immediately after the injury occurred?	Abdominal wall pain or serious intra-abdominal injury
Are you nauseous or have you been vomiting?	Serious intra-abdominal injury
Does eating or drinking make the pain better or worse?	Eating that makes the pain worse may be due to a serious intra-abdominal injury.
Do you have any related (referred) pain to the shoulders or back?	intra-abdominal injury
Do you have any blood in your urine or stools?	Genitourinary or serious intra-abdominal injury
Where is your pain located?	Indicates a possible site of injury
Allergies	
Do you have any known allergies?	This information may be helpful to a physician or paramedic
Medications	
Are you currently taking any medications?	This information may be helpful to a physician or paramedic
Past Medical History	
Do you have any current abdominal conditions or previous abdominal injuries or surgeries?	The current injury could be an aggravation or progression of a previous injury
Last Meal Consumed	
When did you last eat or drink?	Knowledge of any recent meals may be help-
Did you have a full bladder when you were injured?	ful to a physician or paramedic. Also, a full bladder or stomach can indicate a potential for a hollow organ injury
Events Preceding the Injury	
Do you know how you hurt yourself? How much force was applied and where was the abdomen stricken?	This may help to differentiate between the type of abdominal injuries the athlete may have

Table 9-5

Some Signs and Symptoms of a Serious Abdominal Injury Requiring an Immediate Medical Referral[6,8]

Progressive nausea and vomiting
Respiratory symptoms
Continuous local or diffuse abdominal pain
Pain with deep palpation
Blood in urine or stool
Signs of peritoneal irritation:
- Abdominal rigidity
- Involuntary muscle guarding/spasms (the most important sign of peritoneal irritation is muscle guarding)
- Referred tenderness to other parts of the abdomen
- Rebound tenderness (pain with vibration of the abdominal wall and underlying peritoneum)
- Loss of bowel sounds
- Pain referred to the shoulder
- Increased pain with jarring movements such as walking, bouncing, coughing, etc
Signs of a severe male genital traumatic injury:
- Persistent scrotal and/or abdominal pain
- Nausea and vomiting
- Scrotal swelling and/or hematoma
- Scrotal or perineal ecchymosis
- High riding and/or immobile testicle
- Induration (firmness) of scrotum
Abnormally shaped abdomen and/or trunk asymmetry
Moderate to severe ecchymosis:
- Cullen's sign (ecchymosis around the umbilicus—Table 9-10)
- Ecchymosis around the epigastric region (Table 9-10)
- Turner's sign (ecchymosis around the flank—Table 9-11)
- Diffuse abdominal ecchymosis (Table 9-10)
Make an immediate medical referral whenever in doubt regarding the seriousness of the injury

Table 9-6
General Palpation
Gentle abdominal palpation to assess for, and differentiate between, peritoneal irritation and muscle guarding.
- Start palpating away from the injured area.
- Involuntary muscle guarding secondary to peritoneal irritation cannot be decreased by relaxation or distraction (ie, have the athlete breathe deeply or carry on a conversation while palpating the abdomen). Conversely, voluntary muscle guarding from an abdominal wall injury can be diminished by distraction.
- Next, have the athlete lift the head to increase abdominal tension. Peritoneal pain will diminish with palpation when there is an increase in abdominal muscle tension, while abdominal wall pain will increase during palpation due to the presence of an increase in abdominal muscle tension.

Table 9-7
Deep Organ Palpation[13]
Liver:
- Place the athlete in the supine position.
- Place your left hand under the posterior aspect of the lower right ribs and adjacent soft tissues and pull the tissues upward.
- Place your right hand laterally to the right of the rectus muscle, at the inferior costal border.
- Press up and in with the right hand.
- Have the athlete take a deep breath and try to palpate the liver as it descends with inspiration.

Spleen:
- Place the athlete in the supine position.
- The technique is the same as above, except the examiner lifts upward on the left lower ribs and soft tissues.
- Press up and in under the left inferior rib margin and try to palpate the spleen during inspiration.
- This may be performed by having the athlete lie on the contralateral side so that gravity can assist in bringing the spleen forward and medially, making it easier to palpate.

Kidneys (palpation of a right kidney described):
- Place the athlete in the supine position.
- Place your left hand under the right costovertebral angle and lift upward to try to displace the right kidney.
- Place the right hand in the upper quadrant, below the costal margin and lateral to the rectus muscle.
- Have the athlete deeply inspire and pause. When paused, press deep with the right hand and try to capture the kidney. Briefly try to assess its size and tenderness.
- Have the athlete expire the breath and pause. While paused, slowly release the pressure with the right hand and, with the left hand, try to feel the kidney fall back to its normal position.
- Repeat on the left side.
  (It is difficult to palpate the kidneys, especially the left kidney.)

Table 9-8
Special Tests
- Assess for a pelvic fracture by grasping the iliac crests and rocking the pelvis. Also, compress and distract the iliac crests.
- Evaluate for peritoneal irritation by rebound testing the four abdominal quadrants and two regions (depress and quickly release the abdominal wall), shaking/vibrating the abdomen, and have the patient cough. Tests are positive if they provoke pain.
- Percussion of the liver, spleen, and kidneys by making a fist and gently tapping over the areas of the organs.
- Look for blood in the urine and stools (PRN).

Table 9-9

Abdominal Wall Injuries

Condition	Mechanism and General Information	Possible Signs/Symptoms
Muscle injuries (abdominal muscles, iliopsoas, or spinatus/spinal muscles)	1. Caused by overstretching, overuse, a single forceful contraction, blunt trauma, or penetration 2. It is possible to have a concurrent intra-abdominal injury, which may be difficult to assess 3. With severe blunt trauma, the epigastric vessels can rupture, causing a hematoma to develop in the rectus sheath; this requires a physician referral	1. Localized pain and swelling 2. Palpable increased pain during a muscle contraction 3. Voluntary muscle guarding 4. An isolated abdominal wall injury will have no referred pain or systemic signs (nausea, dizziness, dyspnea, etc)

Pelvic injuries (contusions and fractures)	1. Pelvic fractures are due to severe trauma and usually not present in sports injuries
	2. A contusion or hematoma of the margin of the iliac crest that is caused by a direct blow; this is also known as a hip pointer
		1. Pelvic fracture:
		  • Severe pain with pelvic rock test
		  • Blood in urethral meatus or scrotum
		2. Hip pointer:
		  • Localized pain, usually severe
		  • Increased pain with trunk movements and coughing

Solar plexus contusion	See Chapter 8 Requires an abdominal exam to rule out other injuries	See Chapter 8

Table 9-10

Intra-abdominal Injuries

Condition	Mechanism and General Information	Possible Signs/Symptoms
Spleen injury	1. Caused by trauma to the left upper abdominal quadrant or left lower ribs 2. May be associated with a fractured rib 3. An enlarged spleen (ie, from mononucleosis) has an increased risk of injury	1. The pain may be delayed and minor to acute and severe 2. Left shoulder pain may be present due to irritation of the left diaphragm (Kehr's sign) 3. Tenderness over the left upper quadrant, left lower ribs, or left flank progressing to diffuse abdominal pain 4. Pain with percussion and/or deep inspiration 5. Nausea and/or vomiting 6. Anorexia (loss of appetite) 7. If severe, hypovolemic shock and stomach distention
Liver injury	1. Caused by trauma to the right upper abdominal quadrant or right lower ribs. The force can be directed to the front, side, or back 2. Usually associated with significant blood loss 3. Bleeding is usually minimal. Mild injuries usually go undetected. Moderate to severe injuries usually have acute signs	1. Painful mass in right upper quadrant 2. Usually quick onset of peritoneal irritation 3. Hypovolemic shock if severe 4. Pain with percussion 5. Nausea and vomiting 6. Pain may refer to the right shoulder and/or periscapular region

Table 9-10, continued

Condition	Mechanism and General Information	Possible Signs/Symptoms
Small intestine injuries (jejunum and/or ileum)	Caused by a direct force that compresses the bowel against the spinal column or a shearing force in a region where the bowel is fixed to the abdominal cavity	1. Usually no early signs 2. Slowly developing peritoneal irritation 3. Epigastric pain
Small intestine injury (duodenum)	1. Caused by an unexpected blow or a fall on the back 2. The increased pressure of trapped gas causes the duodenum to rupture or tear 3. Associated with injuries to the ribs, spine, liver, or spleen	1. Signs can be initially absent due to the retroperitoneal position of the duodenum 2. Cullen's sign (ecchymosis around the umbilicus, indicative of retroperitoneal bleeding) 3. Vomiting days later if a hematoma develops due to a tear
Mesentery injury	1. Caused by blunt trauma that tears the mesentery	1. A severe injury can cause early peritoneal irritation 2. A minor injury can be asymptomatic for days
Pancreas injury	Caused by a forceful spearing trauma to the mid or upper abdomen such as created by a fist or stick, compressing the pancreas against the spine	1. Usually asymptomatic at first due to its retroperitoneal location 2. Over days, peritoneal irritation will occur over the epigastric abdominal region and spread diffusely over the abdomen 3. Nausea, vomiting, and/or anorexia may develop 4. Pain may be referred to the back 5. Abdominal distention may develop
Stomach injuries	Caused by a blunt injury or blow to the epigastrium	1. Usually an early development of peritoneal irritation due to acid contents of the stomach 2. Epigastric pain with palpation
Large intestine injuries	1. Caused by blunt trauma 2. Associated with other abdominal injuries and can cause bacterial contamination of the abdominal cavity due to rupture of the intestine	Signs of peritoneal irritation are usually delayed; they do not show up until an infection develops
Diaphragm injuries	1. Caused by blunt abdominal trauma 2. The rupture usually occurs on the left side	1. Respiratory distress 2. Collapse of lung 3. Usually severe pain

Table 9-11
Genitourinary Injuries

Condition	Mechanism and General Information	Possible Signs/Symptoms
Kidney injury	1. Caused by direct trauma to the flank or a deceleration injury 2. Usually in the form of a contusion or bruise 3. Renal injury can occur without pain if the damage is isolated within the substance of the kidney 4. Sometimes associated with a lumbar spine or rib fracture	1. Flank pain and tenderness 2. Pain with percussion 3. In severe cases, the development of a mass in the flank and development of hypovolemic shock 4. Guarding 5. Presence of a contusion 6. Dysuria (pain or difficulty with urination) 7. Turner's sign (ecchymosis around the flank, indicative of retroperitoneal bleeding), which develops over hours or days
Bladder injury	1. Caused by blunt trauma to the lower abdomen or a deceleration injury that can cause a contusion or rupture of the bladder 2. A rupture is more likely if the bladder is full	1. Hematuria (blood in the urine, which can be microscopic or grossly visible) 2. Dysuria 3. Lower abdominal pain and tenderness 4. Peritoneal irritation due to urine leakage/loss
Scrotal or testicular contusion	1. Caused by a direct blow that impinges the testicle against the symphysis pubis 2. A hydrocele may develop, which is a cyst that encompasses the testicle due to decreased absorption of the normal tunica vaginalis secretions 3. In severe cases, a rupture of the testicle can develop	1. Immediate nauseating pain 2. Athlete usually drops to the playing surface 3. May have ecchymosis and swelling 4. Palpation of a fluid-filled cyst that encompasses the testicle (hydrocele)
Testicular torsion	Can be caused by a blow to the scrotum or can develop insidiously	1. Acute pain and swelling 2. Nausea and vomiting 3. High-riding testicle
Vulva contusion	A direct blow to the vulva from a straddle-type injury	1. Localized pain 2. A hematoma may develop

References

1. Tucker AM. Abdominal and genital injuries. In: Andrews JR, Clancy WG, Whiteside JA, eds. *On-Field Evaluation and Treatment of Common Athletic Injuries.* St, Louis, Mo: Mosby;1997:63-71.
2. Haycock CE. How I manage abdominal injuries. *Phys Sportsmed.* 1986;14(6):86-99.
3. Bragg LE. Athletic injuries of the thorax and abdomen. In: Mellion M, Walsh W, Shelton G, eds. *The Team Physician's Handbook.* Philadelphia, Pa: Hanley & Belfus; 1990:365-373.
4. Booher J, Thibodeau G. *Athletic Injury Assessment. 3rd ed.* St. Louis, Mo: Mosby; 1994:316-395.
5. Tuttle G. The abdomen. In: Richmond JC, Shahady EJ, eds. *Sports Medicine for Primary Care.* Cambridge, Mass: Blackwell Science; 1996:150-175.
6. Diamond DL. Sports-related abdominal trauma. *Clin Sports Med.* 1989;8:91-99.
7. Colucciello SA, Plotka M. Abdominal trauma: occult injury may be life threatening. *Phys Sportsmed.* 1993;21(6):33-43.
8. Moncure AC, Wilkins EW. Injuries involving the abdomen, viscera, and genitourinary system. In: Vinger PF, Hoerner EF, eds. *Sports Injuries: The Unthwarted Epidemic. 2nd ed.* Littleton, Mass: PSG Publishing Co; 1986:179-187.
9. Bergman RT. Assessing acute abdominal pain. *Phys Sportsmed.* 1996;24(4):72-82.
10. Torg JS, Ramsey-Emrhein JA. Cervical spine and brachial plexus injuries. *Phys Sportsmed.* 1997;25(7):61-88.
11. American Academy of Neurology. Practice parameter: the management of concussion in sports (summary statement). *Neurology.* 1997;48:581-585.
12. Price MB, DeVroom HL. A quick and easy guide to neurological assessment. *J Neurosurg Nurs.* 1985;17:313-320.
13. Bates B, Bickley LS, Hoekelman RA. *A Guide to Physical Examination and History Taking. 6th ed.* Philadelphia, Pa: JB Lippincott Co; 1991:331-400.
14. Bledsoe B, Porter R, Shade B. *Brady Paramedic Emergency Care. 3rd ed.* Upper Saddle River, NJ: Brady Prentice Hall; 1997:469-4970,769-791.
15. Filion DT. Abdominal injuries. *Sports Med Update.* 1997;12(3):12-16.

Bibliography

Amaral JF. Thoracoabdominal injuries in the athlete. *Clin Sports Med.* 1997;16:739-753.

Athletic Training Emergency Care. Course Notebook. Wichita, Kan, April 1997 (c/o DCH Outpatient Services, 809 University Boulevard East, Tuscaloosa, AL 35401).

Boulanger BR, McLellan BA. Blunt abdominal trauma. *Emer Med Clin.* 1996;14:151-171.

Carr S, Troop B, Hurley J, Pennell R. Blunt-trauma carotid artery injury. *Phys Sportsmed.* 1996;24(2):48-54.

Henderson JM, Puffer JC. A case conference: abdominal pain in a football player. *Phys Sportsmed.* 1989;17(8):47-52.

Kenny P. Abdominal pain in athletes. *Clin Sports Med.* 1986;6:885-905.

McAnena OJ, Moore EE, Marx JA. Initial evaluation of the patient with blunt abdominal trauma. *Surg Clin N Amer.* 1990;70:495-515.

Murphy CP, Drez D. Jejunal rupture in a football player. *Am J Sports Med.* 1987;15:184-185.

Perkins RM, Sterling JC. Case conference: left lower chest pain in a collision athlete. *Phys Sportsmed.* 1991;19(3):78-84.

York JP. Sports and the male genitourinary system: genital injuries and sexually transmitted diseases. *Phys Sportsmed.* 1990;18(10):92-100.

Suggested Reading (on Abdominal Evaluations)

Assessment Review Series: Gastrointestinal System. Videotape. Springhouse Corp; 1992.

Assessment Review Series: Reproductive and Urinary Systems. Videotape. Springhouse Corp; 1992.

Bates B, Bickley LS, Hoekelman RA. *A Guide to Physical Examination and History Taking. 6th ed.* Philadelphia, Pa: JB Lippincott Co; 1991:331-400.

Koopermeiners MB. Screening for gastrointestinal system diseases. In: Boissonnault WG, ed. *Examination in Physical Therapy Practice. 2nd ed.* New York, NY: Churchill Livingstone; 1995:101-116.

CHAPTER 10

Heat and Cold Injuries

Athletes can develop heat injuries when they play in a hot and/or humid environment and cold injuries when in a cold environment (a combination of ambient temperature and the wind). However, with improper attire, the weather/environment does not have to be severe for heat and cold injuries to take palace. Mild heat injuries include heat cramps, syncope, and mild heat exhaustion. Mild frostbite is considered a minor form of a cold injury. These mild heat and cold injuries can be managed on the sideline by the sports medicine clinician. All other forms of heat and cold injuries, such as severe heat exhaustion, heat stroke, and hypothermia should be considered severe in nature and require a referral for medical evaluation and treatment.

For the discussion of thermal injuries, the body can be anatomically divided into the shell and the core. The body shell includes the skin, muscles, and extremities. The body core includes the brain, lungs, heart, and abdominal organs. The average core temperature is 98.6°F (37°C). Humans must control their core temperature between the range of 75° to 105°F.[1] The body can lose or gain heat by radiation, conduction, or convection. Additionally, the body can lose heat by evaporation.[2]

The core body temperature should be assessed in collapsed athletes. The most accurate method is to take the rectal temperature. Other methods, such as oral, axillary, or tympanic temperature evaluations, do not correlate to core temperatures in exercising athletes.[3] Axillary temperature may be used in the field if the situation is inappropriate for assessing the rectal temperature or if the clinician feels uncomfortable doing so. However, the clinician should be aware that the axillary temperature may be lower than the actual core temperature.

HEAT INJURIES

It is possible for an athlete to develop an increase in core body temperature over a short period of time, which can rapidly lead to heat illness.[4] Evaporation is the primary means of heat loss. Evaporation occurs due to cutaneous vasodilatation and sweating. In extreme heat, up to 25% of cardiac output passes through the skin. The amount of evaporation that takes place can be limited due to a high level of relative humidity. The relative humidity is the most important factor regarding the effectiveness of evaporation.[2,4] The type of uniform or gear that an athlete wears can also limit evaporation. For example, a football uniform covers about 50% of the athlete's evaporative skin surface and thus can be a factor in developing heat illness.[5] It is also interesting to note that continually drying the skin and/or changing out of a wet uniform hampers evaporative cooling.[2]

The type of uniform or gear that an athlete wears can also limit evaporation. For example, a football uniform covers approximately 50% of the athlete's evaporative skin surface and thus can be a factor in developing heat illness. It is also interesting to note that continually drying the skin and/or changing out of a wet uniform hampers evaporative cooling.

It is beneficial to assess the environmental conditions prior to exercising in the heat.

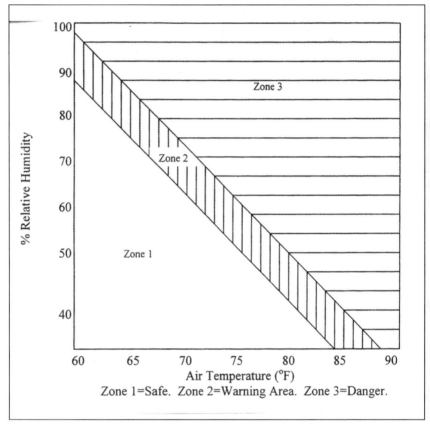

Figure 10-1. Weather guide for the prevention of heat stroke (reprinted with permission from Booher J, Thibodeau G. *Athletic Injury Assessment. 3rd ed.* St. Louis, Mo: Mosby; 1994).

This can be done by using the heat index (combined effect of ambient temperature and humidity), which can be derived by information from a local weather service using a sling psychrometer or a wet bulb thermometer.[4]

It is important for athletes to hydrate prior to and during exercise to try to offset possible dehydration. An acclimatized athlete can loose up to 3 liters of sweat per hour and can reach 12 liters per day (26 pounds). While replacing fluids during exercise, the body can only empty 800 mL per hour from the stomach. Therefore, it is impossible to replenish all of the fluid lost. Thus, dehydration can progress during exercise in hot and humid environments, even if the athlete is rehydrating during exercise.[2] An athlete should try to consume 400 to 800 mL of fluid 15 to 20 minutes before exercising.[2,6] Fluids should also be ingested during practice and play. Fluid absorption rates can be increased if the stomach is already partially filled with fluid.[2,7] Additionally, the body looses 2.3 to 3.4 grams of sodium per liter of sweat. When exercising in a hot and humid environment for a period of time, it is possible for an athlete to loose 13 to 17 grams of sodium per day.[2] Therefore, placing an extra amount of salt on food may be beneficial to athletes who exercise in hot and humid environments. Eating a well-balanced diet will help to provide the athlete with important minerals and fluids to replenish those lost during sweating.

The different types of heat illness are all caused by exercise in a hot and humid environment. The signs and symptoms of different types of heat illness overlap to some extent.

	Ambient Temperature, °F**															
	40	35	30	25	20	15	10	5	0	-5	-10	-15	-20	-25	-30	
	Equivalent Temperature, °F															
Calm	40	35	30	25	20	15	10	5	0	-5	-10	-15	-20	-25	-30	Calm
5	37	33	27	21	16	12	6	1	-5	-11	-15	-20	-26	-31	-35	5
10	28	21	16	9	4	-2	-9	-15	-21	-27	-33	-38	-46	-52	-58	10
15	22	16	11	1	-5	-11	-18	-25	-36	-40	-45	-51	-58	-65	-70	15
20	18	12	3	-4	-10	-17	-25	-32	-39	-46	-53	-60	-67	-76	-81	20
25	16	7	0	-7	-15	-22	-29	-37	-44	-52	-59	-67	-74	-83	-89	25
30	13	5	-2	-11	-18	-26	-33	-41	-48	-56	-63	-70	-79	-87	-94	30
35	11	3	-4	-13	-20	-27	-35	-43	-49	-60	-67	-72	-82	-90	-98	35
40*	10	1	-6	-15	-21	-29	-37	-45	-53	-62	-69	-76	-85	-94	-101	40*
	Little Danger					Danger					Great Danger					

*Convective heat loss at wind speeds above 40 mph have little additional effect on body cooling.
** °C = 0.556 (°F −32)

Figure 10-2. The wind chill index (reprinted with permission from McArdle WD, Katch FI, Katch VL. *Exercise Physiology: Energy, Nutrition, and Human Performance.* Philadelphia, Pa; 1986).

Thus, it can be difficult to differentiate the types of heat illnesses.[2] Also, realize that when one athlete develops a heat illness, the conditions are present for other athletes to develop heat illnesses as well.[6]

Risk Factors for Developing Heat Illness

- Age: heat illness occurs more in children and the elderly.
- Illness: any acute illness that causes a fever or fluid loss (diarrhea and/or vomiting) can predispose an athlete to developing a heat illness. Chronic illnesses such as cardiac disease or eating disorders can also predispose someone for developing a heat illness.
- Gender: males have more incidence of heat illness than do females.
- Body type: obese athletes, or those in poor physical conditions, are more likely to develop a heat illness.
- Environmental conditions: Hot, humid, and windless days predispose athletes to develop heat illness. Athletes that are nonacclimatized or in poor physical condition are more prone to heat illness.
- Inappropriate clothing: athletes that are overdressed or wearing nonbreathable materials are at greater risk of developing a heat illness.
- Use of alcohol or nonprescription drugs: alcohol increases dehydration, decreases cardiac output, and can cause electrolyte disturbances. Additionally, cocaine and amphetamines increase physical activity and decrease awareness of fatigue. All of the above can lead to heat illness.
- An athlete who has suffered a previous heat illness may have some permanent damage to the thermoregulatory system and is thus more prone to developing a future heat illness.[4]

COLD ILLNESS

The coldness of an environment depends on the ambient temperature and the wind.[2] For example, exposure to a 65°F environment for 3 hours can cause hypothermia if there are high wind chill and wetness factors.[8] Knowledge of the wind chill index would be helpful for the sports medicine clinician who is covering outdoor winter sports. Remember that there is a wind chill effect if a moving athlete (eg, snow skier, ice skater) is going in the same direction (which would decrease the wind chill) or opposite direction of the wind (which would increase the wind chill).[2,9] Also, keep in mind that temperatures below or above freezing can cause frostbite/localized cold injuries.[1]

It is best to dress with layered clothing when exercising in a cold environment. The layer next to the skin should be a fabric that can wick moisture from the body (eg, wool). The outer layer should be windproof and preferably breathable (eg, GoreTex). It is also important to wear gloves, cap, and some neck and facial covering.

Risk Factors for Developing Hypothermia

- Wet clothing or improper attire. Wet clothing loses up to 90% of its insulating properties.[2]
- Being in a dehydrated state.
- Malnutrition: in a state of malnutrition, there is less energy for muscle contractions and lack of heat production from digestion.
- Alcohol consumption: the vasodilatation that occurs from alcohol consumption leads to increased heat loss.
- Physical exhaustion: with fatigue there is a decrease in muscle contractions, which leads to less development of metabolic heat.
- Environmental conditions: increased ambient temperatures, humidity, and altitude can create an environment that makes athletes more susceptible to cold injuries.
- Extreme ages: children and the elderly have an increased risk of developing a cold injury.
- Medication use that can increase heat loss.
- Body type: with leanness/low levels of body fat, there is less insulation from the cold.
- Some medical conditions, such as diabetes or thyroid disease.

EVALUATION OF HEAT OR COLD INJURIES

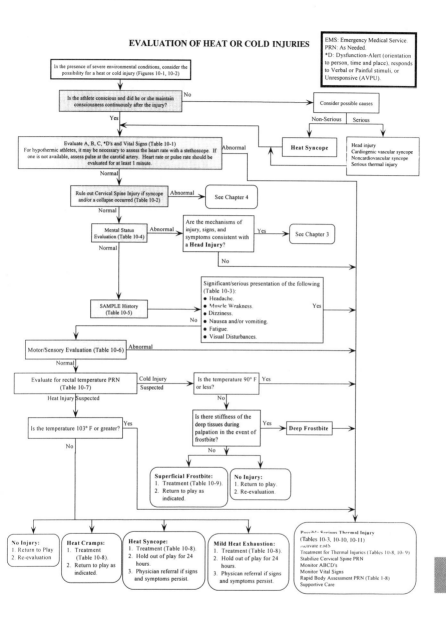

EMS: Emergency Medical Service.
PRN: As Needed.
*D: Dysfunction-Alert (orientation to person, time and place), responds to Verbal or Painful stimuli, or Unresponsive (AVPU).

In the presence of severe environmental conditions, consider the possibility for a heat or cold injury (Figures 10-1, 10-2)

Is the athlete conscious and did he or she maintain consciousness continuously after the injury?

No → Consider possible causes

Non-Serious → Heat Syncope

Serious → Head injury / Cardiogenic vascular syncope / Noncardiovascular syncope / Serious thermal injury

Yes

Evaluate A, B, C, *D's and Vital Signs (Table 10-1)
For hypothermic athletes, it may be necessary to assess the heart with a stethoscope. If one is not available, assess pulse at the carotid artery. Heart rate or pulse rate should be evaluated for at least 1 minute.

Abnormal →

Normal

Rule out Cervical Spine Injury if syncope and/or a collapse occurred (Table 10-2)

Abnormal → See Chapter 4

Normal

Mental Status Evaluation (Table 10-4)

Abnormal → Are the mechanisms of injury, signs, and symptoms consistent with a Head Injury?

Yes → See Chapter 3

No

Normal

SAMPLE History (Table 10-5)

Significant/serious presentation of the following (Table 10-3):
● Headache.
● Muscle Weakness.
● Dizziness.
● Nausea and/or vomiting.
● Fatigue.
● Visual Disturbances.

Yes →

No

Motor/Sensory Evaluation (Table 10-6)

Abnormal →

Normal

Evaluate for rectal temperature PRN (Table 10-7)

Cold Injury Suspected → Is the temperature 90° F or less?

Yes →

No

Heat Injury Suspected

Is the temperature 103° F or greater?

Yes →

No

Is there stiffness of the deep tissues during palpation in the event of frostbite?

Yes → Deep Frostbite →

No

Superficial Frostbite:
1. Treatment (Table 10-9).
2. Return to play as indicated.

No Injury:
1. Return to play.
2. Re-evaluation.

No Injury:
1. Return to Play
2. Re-evaluation

Heat Cramps:
1. Treatment (Table 10-8).
2. Return to play as indicated.

Heat Syncope:
1. Treatment (Table 10-8).
2. Hold out of play for 24 hours.
3. Physician referral if signs and symptoms persist.

Mild Heat Exhaustion:
1. Treatment (Table 10-8).
2. Hold out of play for 24 hours.
3. Physician referral if signs and symptoms persist.

Possible Serious Thermal Injury
(Tables 10-3, 10-10, 10-11)
Activate EMS
Treatment for Thermal Injuries (Tables 10-8, 10-9)
Stabilize Cervical Spine PRN
Monitor ABCD's
Monitor Vital Signs
Rapid Body Assessment PRN (Table 1-8)
Supportive Care

Table 10-1

Vital Signs—Possible Findings in the Presence of a Thermal Injury*

Sign	Heat Illness	Cold Illness
Pulse rate	Tachycardia	Bradycardia
Respiration rate	Tachypnea	Dyspnea; decreased rate and depth
Blood pressure	Possible hypotension	Possible hypotension
Skin color	Can be red or ash and gray	Pale, gray, waxy, or purple (if thawing after frostbite or in late hypothermia)
Pupils	May be fixed and constricted	Can be dilated

*See Table 1-2 for normal data

Table 10-2

Some Signs and Symptoms of a Significant Cervical Spine Injury[4,10]

- Involuntary loss of bowel and/or bladder control
- Cervical pain without movement
- Pain with palpation over the posterior or anterior cervical spine
- Rigid muscle spasms of the anterior and/or posterior neck muscles
- Deformity detected by palpation or the presence of a wryneck (abnormal neck position usually including flexion, rotation, and side bending)
- Decreased cervical spine mobility with pain
- Persistent burning, weakness, tingling, or numbness in any extremity

Table 10-3

Some Signs and Symptoms Requiring an Immediate Physician Referral

Hyperthermia
- Altered level of consciousness
- Impaired mental status
- Core temperature of 104° F or greater
- Ataxia (irregular and poorly coordinated muscle contraction)
- Oligurea (diminished urine output in relation to the amount of fluid intake)
- Cessation of sweating with hot and dry skin
- Convulsive seizures
- Constricted pupils
- Nausea and/or vomiting
- Severe fatigue
- Muscle cramping
- Visual disturbances
- Collapse without warning

Hypothermia
- Altered level of consciousness
- Impaired mental status
- Core temperature below 95°F
- Ataxia/clumsy
- Flattened affect/apathetic
- Paradoxical undressing (removing protective clothing)
- Muscular rigidity
- No shivering
- Make an immediate medical referral whenever in doubt of the seriousness of the injury

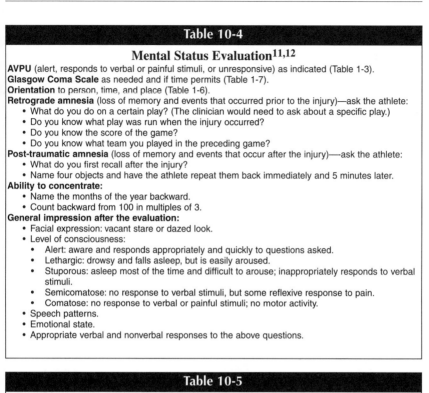

Table 10-4

Mental Status Evaluation[11,12]

AVPU (alert, responds to verbal or painful stimuli, or unresponsive) as indicated (Table 1-3).
Glasgow Coma Scale as needed and if time permits (Table 1-7).
Orientation to person, time, and place (Table 1-6).
Retrograde amnesia (loss of memory and events that occurred prior to the injury)—ask the athlete:
- What do you do on a certain play? (The clinician would need to ask about a specific play.)
- Do you know what play was run when the injury occurred?
- Do you know the score of the game?
- Do you know what team you played in the preceding game?

Post-traumatic amnesia (loss of memory and events that occur after the injury)—ask the athlete:
- What do you first recall after the injury?
- Name four objects and have the athlete repeat them back immediately and 5 minutes later.

Ability to concentrate:
- Name the months of the year backward.
- Count backward from 100 in multiples of 3.

General impression after the evaluation:
- Facial expression: vacant stare or dazed look.
- Level of consciousness:
  - Alert: aware and responds appropriately and quickly to questions asked.
  - Lethargic: drowsy and falls asleep, but is easily aroused.
  - Stuporous: asleep most of the time and difficult to arouse; inappropriately responds to verbal stimuli.
  - Semicomatose: no response to verbal stimuli, but some reflexive response to pain.
  - Comatose: no response to verbal or painful stimuli; no motor activity.
- Speech patterns.
- Emotional state.
- Appropriate verbal and nonverbal responses to the above questions.

Table 10-5

SAMPLE History

Question	Interpretation
Symptoms	
Do you have any of the following symptoms: Headaches, weakness, dizziness, thirsty, nausea, or visual disturbances?	These are all symptoms of a thermal injury
Allergies	
Do you have any known allergies?	Some signs and symptoms of a thermal injury can resemble an anaphylactic reaction. Also, knowledge of known allergies can be helpful to a physician or paramedic
Medications	
Are you currently taking any medications?	Specific medications can contribute to heat illness. Also, this information may be helpful to a physician or paramedic
Past Medical History	
Have you ever had a heat illness before?	Having had a previous heat injury predisposes someone to developing another heat injury
Last Meal Consumed	
When did you last eat or drink?	Try to assess the hydration status of the athlete by asking about fluid intake prior to and during the exercise bout
Events Preceding the Injury	
Did you receive a blow to the head before your symptoms started?	Mental status changes that occur with an apparent heat illness may actually be due to a head injury
Do you remember what happened just prior to the onset of your signs and symptoms?	This is a possible test for retrograde amnesia. Also, this may help to differentiate between the type of thermal injury the athlete may have

Table 10-6

Motor-Sensory Evaluation*

Motor Tests (for dysfunctions of the cerebellum, spinal cord, peripheral nerves, and/or cerebrum/upper motor neurons):
- Normal muscle tone: Palpation and passive range of motion to test for rigidity or flaccidness.
- Test strength of major muscle groups.

Sensation Tests (for dysfunctions of the spinal cord, peripheral nerves, and/or cerebrum/higher sensory pathways):
- Test light touch sensation of extremities and trunk.

Reflex Tests (for dysfunctions of the spinal cord, peripheral nerves, muscles, and/or cerebrum/higher pathways):
- Deep tendon reflexes: biceps, brachioradialis, triceps, quadriceps, and Achilles tendons.

Coordination Tests (for dysfunctions of the motor, cerebellar, vestibular, and/or sensory systems):
- Romberg's test: have the athlete stand with the feet together, hands at sides, and eyes open. Then have the athlete close the eyes. The test is positive if the patient sways back and forth or falls to one side.
- Finger to nose test: with the eyes closed, have the athlete touch his or her nose with alternating forefingers and with increasing speed. The test is positive if the nose is not consistently touched.
- Heel to knee test: in supine, have the athlete alternatively touch the ground and contralateral knee with the heel. The test is positive if the patella is not consistently touched.

*Primarily assessed in this chapter for a lesion to the motor or sensory systems of the brain[4,13]

Table 10-7

Evaluation of Rectal Temperature

1. Protect the athlete's privacy by covering him or her with a thin sheet (hyperthermic) or blanket (hypothermic) if available.
2. Insert the thermometer 5 cm beyond the anal sphincter.
3. Evaluate the temperature 5 to 10 minutes after placement of the thermometer.

Table 10-8

Treatment of Heat Illness

Heat Syncope
- Place in a cool, shaded area with the athlete supine and feet elevated
- Rest
- Fluid intake may be helpful

Heat Cramps
- Slowly apply a sustained stretch to the contracted muscle
- Apply ice to the contracted muscle
- Massage the contracted muscle
- Drink water (a hypotonic solution of 1 teaspoon of salt to 1 quart of cold water or two 10-grain salt tablets crushed in 1 liter of water)

Heat Exhaustion
- Remove from the hot environment into a cool, shaded area
- Place supine and elevate feet
- Cool the athlete by sponging or toweling with cool water, fanning, and/or placing ice bags around the great vessels (place them around the lateral neck, axilla, groin, and even the head)
- Give fluids if athlete is conscious. Continue hydration until pre-exercise body weight is achieved and polyurea is present
- For mild heat exhaustion (core temperature less than 103°F, no alteration in mental status or level of consciousness, no ataxia), remove from activity for 24 hours and observe for residual weight loss
- For severe heat exhaustion (core temperature of 103°F or greater, altered mental status or level of consciousness, and/or ataxia), activate EMS
- Activate EMS if unsure of the severity of the heat exhaustion

Heatstroke
- Activate EMS
- Remove from the hot environment and remove clothing
- Cool the body as stated above
- Have the athlete drink cold water, if conscious
- Stop cooling when the core temperature stabilizes at 102°F to avoid overcooling
- Continue to assess core temperature every 5 to 10 minutes to check for a rebound effect occurs. If so, continue cooling efforts

Table 10-9
Treatment of Cold Illness

Superficial Frostbite
- Can be thawed on the field, but it is best to take the athlete to a warm shelter
- Place a warm object or hand on the injured area or place the injured area in a warm environment (eg, inside a warm jacket or armpit)

Deep Frostbite
- Do not thaw if there is a risk of refreezing
- It is best treated in a hospital setting. Keep the part frozen during transport
- It is best to rapidly warm the injured tissue (eg, in warm water between 104o and 108o F) if access to a hospital is limited. Once rewarmed, place sterile bandages over the involved area and refer to a physician as soon as possible

Mild Hypothermia
- Remove the athlete from the cold environment to a shelter
- Evaluate rectal temperature
- Activate EMS
- Avoid any jostling movements, which could cause ventricular fibrillation
- Replace wet clothing with dry clothing
- Have the athlete lay supine. Do not allow sitting, standing, or walking until rewarmed
- Insulate the athlete with blankets. One or two other people can lie next to the athlete for insulation. It is best to apply hot water bottles, heating pads, or electric blanket only to the trunk.
- Hot drinks may be beneficial if the athlete can swallow
- Do not have the athlete exercise to warm up

Moderate to Severe Hypothermia
- Activate EMS. Since the athlete is in somewhat of a hibernated state, it is best to withhold treatment until he or she reaches a hospital. There is controversy regarding the appropriateness of treating this condition in the field. This even includes administering CPR, which can cause asystole (cardiac standstill). It is best treated in a hospital by trained individuals
- Treat the athlete gently to avoid jostling or bumps, which may lead to ventricular fibrillation
- Remember that patients with severe hypothermia have been revived after up to 3 hours of asystole. If a severely hypothermic athlete has no pulse, there is still a chance of survival[9]

Table 10-10

Heat Illnesses

Condition	Mechanism and General Information	Possible Signs/Symptoms
Heat edema	1. Swelling of hands and feet 2. Usually occurs during acclimatization	Mild swelling of hands and feet
Heat syncope	1. Caused by decreased vasomotor tone and venous pooling that occurs when exercising in the heat 2. Blood pools in the periphery, usually when standing after cessation of a bout of exercise 3. Heat syncope can occur from just standing in the heat prior to exercise	1. Fainting, especially after stopping exercise 2. Usually brief prodromal symptoms of dizziness and light-headedness 3. No increase in core temperature 4. Quick return of normal mental and physiological state
Militia rubra (prickly heat)	1. A rash that occurs on skin covered with clothing 2. The rash is due to clogging of pores from the formation of a keratin plug and/or swelling of the sweat glands themselves.	Development of a red rash on the clothed skin of the athlete
Heat cramps	1. There are two theories on the cause. One is that it is from de-hydration. The second theory is that it is due to a chronic sodium depletion that is compounded by an acute sodium loss via profuse sweating 2. Usually occurs in acclimatized athletes 3. The muscles in the lower extremities are primarily affected, including the calf, hamstrings, and quadriceps; however, the ab-dominal and intercostal muscles can also be affected 4. Usually the cramp appears to move about in the muscle since only a few muscle fibers are involved at one time 5. Heat cramps can lead to heat exhaustion	1. Involuntary muscle contractions 2. Sudden onset 3. Muscle cramps can occur during or after exercise 4. Usually extremely painful 5. The athlete does not have any changes in mental status 6. The skin is wet and warm 7. Temperature, pulse, and respiration rates are normal or slightly elevated

Heat exhaustion	1. There are two causes: the first is hypovolemia due to excessive water depletion. The second is due to sodium depletion
	2. Usually heat exhaustion is due to a combination of water and sodium depletion
	3. If not treated, it can lead to heat stroke
	4. Heat exhaustion develops in unacclimatized athletes during hard practice sessions early in the season
	5. Heat exhaustion may resemble a viral infection or food poisoning
	6. A good way to avoid heat exhaustion is to weigh athletes before and after practice to assess weight loss, which correlates to fluid loss
	  • With a 1% loss of body weight, dehydration begins
	  • With a 2% loss, thermoregulation is affected
		1. Profuse sweating, making the skin cool and clammy
		2. Pale or gray skin color
		3. Headache
		4. Muscle weakness
		5. Thirst
		6. Dizziness
		7. Nausea and/or vomiting
		8. Fatigue
		9. Ataxia (irregular and poorly coordinated muscle contraction)
		10. Diarrhea
		11. Piloerection ("goose flesh")
		12. Oligurea (diminished urine output in relation to the amount of fluid intake)

Table 10-10, continued

Condition	Mechanism and General Information	Possible Signs/Symptoms
	• With a 3% loss, performance is affected • With a 4% to 5% loss, muscular work declines by 20% to 30% 7. Heat exhaustion may be further divided into mild and severe degrees • Mild heat exhaustion includes a core temperature less than 103°F, no alteration in mental status or level of consciousness, and no ataxia • Severe heat exhaustion includes core temperature of 103°F or greater, altered mental status or level of consciousness, and/or ataxia	13. Mental status is normal to slightly impaired 14. Body temperature is normal or above normal (can reach 104°F) 15. Tachypnea and possible hyperventilation 16. Tachycardia 17. Hypotension 18. Possible unconsciousness 19. Possible heat cramps 20. Visual disturbances 21. May collapse without warning
Heatstroke	1. Due to failure of the thermoregulatory system, leading to a severe increase in body temperature 2. A true medical emergency; there is a 50% to 75% fatality rate 3. Heatstroke can lead to circulatory collapse, central nervous system (CNS) dysfunction, and death 4. Heatstroke is the second most common cause of death in athletes 5. It is the length of time that the core temperature is elevated, not the absolute rise in core temperature, that is the prognosticating factor 6. Fifty percent of heatstroke victims have a cessation of sweating, while the other 50% are profusely sweating 7. An elevated core temperature of 105°F and a change in alertness and mental status are the primary differences between heat exhaustion and heatstroke	1. The sweating mechanism may be shut down in the late phase, which would cause the skin to be hot and dry and look red 2. However, in exertion heat heatstroke, the athlete may be profusely sweating. In this case the skin may be wet, cool, and look gray 3. Core temperature above 105°F 4. Loss of consciousness that may be followed by a spontaneous return of consciousness 5. While unconscious, there may be a loss of bowel and bladder function 6. Progressive CNS changes: confusion, disorientation, agitation/irritability, hysterical behavior, delirium, and coma 7. May collapse without warning or may have prodromal symptoms of dizziness, weakness, and nausea 8. Convulsive seizures may occur, especially during cooling 9. Tachypnea and possible hyperventilation 10. The hyperventilation can cause tingling in the hands, feet, and around the mouth 11. Pulse is initially rapid and full, and progresses to rapid and weak 12. Hypotension 13. Pupils may be constricted 14. Ataxia to inability to use legs

Table 10-11

Cold Illnesses

Condition	Mechanism and General Information	Possible Signs/Symptoms
Chilblains (perino)	1. A neurocirculatory condition that causes skin lesions 2. Caused by moderately cool temperatures and high humidity 3. Usually a chronic condition	1. Edematous, red, and tender skin lesions 2. Itching 3. Chronic inflammation
Superficial frostbite (frostnip)	1. Freezing of the outer layer of the skin 2. All degrees of frostbite most commonly affect the face, ears, nose, fingers, toes, and sometimes penis 3. Use of tobacco or wearing restrictive clothes increases the risk of developing mild to severe frostbite	1. Burning feeling, followed by numbness 2. Gray or pale skin 3. Deeper tissues are soft and pliable 4. Red, sensitive, and swollen after thawing
Deep frostbite	1. Freezing of the deeper tissue layers 2. After thawing, the skin appears purple; there is also severe pain, blistering, and possible gangrene	1. The involved area is initially subjectively cold but is replaced by a feeling of numbness 2. The skin looks pale and waxy 3. Palpable firm and rigid deep tissues 4. Blisters occur after thawing
Mild hypothermia	Occurs when the core body temperature is between 90° and 95°F	1. Shivering 2. Appears clumsy 3. Stumbles 4. Amnesia 5. Slurred speech 6. Confused 7. Apathetic 8. Desire for sleep
Moderate to severe hypothermia	1. Occurs when the core body temperature is below 90°F 2. It may be difficult to assess the pulse 3. Death usually occurs below 78°F	1. No shivering 2. Flattened effect 3. Paradoxical undressing (removing protective clothing) 4. Muscular rigidity 5. Jerky movements 6. Coma 7. Impairment of consciousness

References

1. Bowman WD. Safe exercise in the cold and cold injuries. In: Mellion MB, Walsh WM, Shelton GL, eds. *The Team Physician's Handbook*. Philadelphia, Pa: Hanley & Belfus; 1990:70-77.
2. McArdle WD, Katch FI, Katch VL. *Exercise Physiology: Energy, Nutrition, and Human Performance*. Philadelphia, Pa: Lea and Febiger;1986:441-466.
3. Roberts WO. Assessing core temperature in collapsed athletes. *Phys Sportsmed*. 1994;22(8):49-55.
4. Booher J, Thibodeau G. *Athletic Injury Assessment. 3rd ed*. St. Louis, Mo: Mosby;1994:118-145,266-289, 316-353.
5. Mathews DK, et al. Physiological responses during exercise and recovery in a football uniform. *J Appl Physiol*. 1969;26:611-615.
6. Cobb CH, Hrabal TL, Sherker RS. Environmental injuries. In: Baker CL, ed. *The Hughston Clinic Sports Medicine Book*. Baltimore, Md: Williams & Wilkins; 1995:45-55.
7. Montain SJ, Maughan RJ, Sawka MN. Fluid replacement strategies for exercise in hot weather. *Athletic Therapy Today*. 1996;1(4):24-27.
8. Lambert SD. Environmental conditions. In: Sanders B, ed. *Sports Physical Therapy*. Norwalk, Conn; 1990:61-78.
9. Thein LA. Environmental conditions affecting the athlete. *JOSPT*. 1995:158-171.
10. American Academy of Neurology. Practice parameter: the management of concussion in sports (summary statement). *Neurology*. 1997;48:581-585.
11. Price MB, DeVroom HL. A quick and easy guide to neurological assessment. *J Neurosurg Nurs*. 1985;17:313-320.
12. Bates B, Bickley LS, Hoekelman RA. *A Guide to Physical Examination and History Taking. 6th ed*. Philadelphia, Pa: JB Lippincott Co; 1991:491-554.

Bibliography

Bernard TE. Risk management for preventing heat illness in athletes. *Athletic Therapy Today*. 1996;1(4):19-21.
Costrini AM, Pitt HA, Gustafson AB, Uddin DE. Cardiovascular and metabolic manifestations of heat stroke and severe heat exhaustion. *Am J Med*. 1979;66:296-302.
Cushner GB, Cushner FD. Fluid balance. In: Scuderi GR, McCann PD, Bruno PJ, eds. *Sports Medicine: Principles of Primary Care*. St. Louis, Mo; 1997:568-577.
DeBenedette V. Sweat: up close and personal. *Phys Sportsmed*. 1991;19(4):103-107.
Hubbard RW, Armstrong LE. Hyperthermia: new thoughts on an old problem. *Phys Sportsmed*. 1989;17(6):97-113.
Knochel JP. Management of heat conditions. *Athletic Therapy Today*. 1996;1(4):30-34.
Mellion MB, Shelton GL. Safe exercise in the heat and heat injuries. In: Mellion MB, Walsh WM, Shelton GL, eds. *The Team Physician's Handbook*. Philadelphia, Pa: Hanley & Belfus; 1990:59-69.
Roberts WO. Managing heatstroke: on site cooling. *Phys Sportsmed*. 1992;20(5):17-28.
Sandor RP. Heat illness: on-site diagnosis and cooling. *Phys Sportsmed*. 1997;25(6):35-40.
Shapiro Y, Seidman DS. Field and clinical observations of exertional heat stroke patients. *Med Sci Sport Exer*. 1990;22(1):6-14.
Thorton JS. Hypothermia shouldn't freeze out cold-weather athletes. *Phys Sportsmed*. 1990;18:109-113.
Torg JS, Ramsey-Emrhein JA. Cervical spine and brachial plexus injuries. *Phys Sportsmed*. 1997;25(7):61-88.
Williams DS. Heat problems and dehydration. In: Andrews JR, Clancy WG, Whiteside JA, eds. *On-Field Evaluation and Treatment of Common Athletic Injuries*. St. Louis, Mo: Mosby; 1997:72-77.

CHAPTER 11

General Medical Problems

The purposes of this chapter are to briefly list and discuss some common medical problems that may occur in athletes. The basic topics include shock, diabetes, nontraumatic chest pain, nontraumatic dyspnea, exercise-induced allergies, and nontraumatic abdominal pain. Some topics are discussed in more depth due to their more frequent occurrence and/or their more emergent nature.

SHOCK

Tissue perfusion is dependent on three components, including the heart, blood, and blood vessels. A dysfunction of any one of these components can cause shock.[1] Although there are several types of shock, they all have the same underlying pathophysiology that leads to inadequate tissue perfusion and decreased oxygen delivery to cells.[1] Shock should be suspected when evaluating any injury.

There are three stages of shock:[1]

- Compensated stage: the body's initial response to inadequate tissue perfusion includes an increased heart rate and contraction strength to increase cardiac output, and vasoconstriction to increase blood pressure. Common signs of this stage include tachycardia, strong pulse, decreased skin perfusion, and slight changes in mental status.
- Decompensated stage: if inadequate tissue perfusion persists, the blood pressure will fall. Heart rate will increase, but contractile strength will decrease; this will lead to decreased cardiac output. A combination of the above will cause the blood-flow to stagnate. Signs of this stage include decreased capillary refill time and a rapid and thready (weak) pulse. Mental status changes will occur initially, including agitation and restlessness, progressing to confusion and coma.
- Irreversible shock: if inadequate perfusion cannot be compensated for, the cells will die. This will lead to tissue death, organ death, and eventually death of the athlete. Even if revived from this stage, the athlete may die from end organ failure of the respiratory, liver, or renal systems.

Despite the type of shock an athlete has, treatment of shock should include the following:[1-3]

- Activate EMS
- If the athlete has anaphylactic shock, administer epinephrine if available
- Maintain a clear airway
- Control bleeding PRN
- Remove restricting clothing that may interfere with circulation or respiration
- Elevate lower extremities, unless there is a head, spinal, pulmonary, or abdominal injury
- Keep the athlete supine
- Splint fractures PRN

- Prevent loss of body heat, but do not overheat
- Do not give anything to eat or drink
- Monitor and record vital signs

Depending on the individual athlete, insect stings can lead to anaphylactic shock. Treatment of an insect sting should include the following:[4]

- Remove the stinger by flicking it out of the skin with the edge of a knife, credit card, or similar object. Do not use tweezers, as this may cause more venom to be squeezed into the skin
- Clean the skin with soap and water or an antiseptic solution
- Apply ice
- A topical agent may be helpful to denature the venom, such as meat tenderizer or baking soda
- Use anti-inflammatory agents such as a nonsteroidal anti-inflammatory drug or ointment

DIABETES

Individuals with type I diabetes (insulin dependent) have a higher risk of developing diabetic emergencies than do athletes with type II diabetes (noninsulin dependent).[5] Remember that insulin requirements are reduced during exercise since the muscles can increase glucose uptake without great need of insulin.[6]

The risk of insulin shock can be reduced by the following:[5-7]

- Decreasing insulin and/or choosing injection sites that are in a muscle that will not be very active during the individual's sporting event.
- Consuming more carbohydrates before, during, and after exercise.
- The athlete must know the type of insulin being taken (short-, intermediate-, or long-acting) and when it is peaking in relation to their exercise schedule.
- Monitoring blood glucose levels, insulin, dietary intake, and exercise intensity for months in order to predict the need for insulin and food. Every athlete reacts differently to insulin, food intake, and exercise. Therefore, this is somewhat of a trial and error process.
- Maintain a state of hydration.
- Exercise in the mornings when there is a decreased risk of developing hypoglycemia.

NONTRAUMATIC CHEST PAIN

Nontraumatic chest pain can be divided into different categories, including cardiac, musculoskeletal, gastrointestinal (GI), pulmonary, and psychogenic.[8,9] Cardiac and pulmonary causes are the most medically serious. Chest pain due to cardiac causes is rare in adolescent athletes. In general, an athlete who has chest pain due to a cardiac disorder may present with some of the following symptoms: syncope, near syncope, palpitations, malaise, classic angina pectoris, dyspnea, and/or undue fatigue.[10,11] In adolescents, the most common pulmonary causes of chest pain are asthma, pneumonia, hyperventilation, and spontaneous pneumothorax.[10] A physician should evaluate all nontraumatic chest pain (with the exception of a controlled asthma attack).

NONTRAUMATIC DYSPNEA

The different categories of nontraumatic dyspnea include airway obstruction; diffuse lung disease; chest wall abnormalities; pulmonary embolism; cardiogenic, psychogenic, or noncardiogenic pulmonary edema; anemia; and obesity.[12] A physician should evaluate all nontraumatic dyspnea (with the exception of a controlled asthma attack, a mild respiratory infection, or after the successful removal of a foreign body without secondary problems).

EXERCISE-INDUCED ALLERGIES

The different categories of exercise-induced allergies include exercise-induced bronchospasm, urticaria, and anaphylaxis. Exercise-induced bronchospasm is relatively common, while urticaria and anaphylaxis are rare.

NONTRAUMATIC ABDOMINAL PAIN

The GI system is divided into the upper and lower GI systems. The upper GI system includes the esophagus, stomach, and duodenum. The lower GI system includes the distal small intestine, colon, and rectum.[1] Symptoms of upper GI problems include nausea, hematemesis, dark stools, bloating, gas, and abdominal pain. Symptoms of lower GI problems include cramping, diarrhea, and bloody stools.[1,13] The complaint of abdominal pain can be the symptom of a serious surgical problem or a relatively benign problem.[14]

The following signs and symptoms suggest a possible severe problem that requires an emergent medical referral:[14]

- Pain that is sudden in onset, severe, progressive, and continuous
- Pain that lasts more than 6 hours
- Pain that is located away from the umbilicus and/or changes in location (appears to spread due to peritoneal irritation)
- Pain that begins during nighttime or during inactivity
- The initial symptom is pain, followed by possible nausea, vomiting, and anorexia.
- Fever is present, without the presence of chills
- Constipation (no passage of stools or gas)
- Increased pain with coughing, sneezing, or bouncing (caused by peritoneal irritation, see Chapter 9)

The following signs and symptoms suggest a less severe problem and require a medical referral but not on an emergency basis:[14]

- Gradual-onset pain, mild to moderate in intensity, and is intermittent
- Pain that decreases or resolves in 6 hours
- Pain that is located near the umbilicus
- The pain is developed near or during a bout of exercise or eating
- Nausea, vomiting, and anorexia develop first, followed by pain
- The athlete may have fever and chills.
- A bowel movement that may temporarily decrease the pain.

Table 11-1

Shock[1-3]

Condition	Mechanism and General Information	Possible Signs/Symptoms
General shock	Includes all different types of shock listed to left	1. Rapid and strong pulse, progressing to a rapid and weak pulse 2. Pale, moist, and cool skin 3. Shallow, rapid respiration 4. Diaphoresis (excessive perspiration) 5. Agitation and restlessness 6. Nausea and vomiting 7. Hypotension 8. Confusion 9. Dilated pupils 10. Coma 11. Death
Hypovolemic shock	1. Due to fluid (plasma) loss 2. Some causes include hemorrhage, dehydration, diabetic coma, and burns	
Respiratory shock	Due to impaired breathing, causing impaired oxygen exchange in the lungs	
Neurogenic shock	1. Loss of sympathetic control to the blood vessels, leading to vaso-dilatation 2. Causes include spinal cord injury, central nervous system injury, and insulin shock	
Vasovagal shock	1. The common "faint" 2. See Chapter 2 for vasovagal syncope	
Cardiogenic shock	Caused by inadequate heart function	
Anaphylactic shock	A severe allergic reaction that can be caused by an insect sting, ingested or inhaled substance, exercise, or injected medication or antitoxin	Specific signs and symptoms of anaphylactic shock: 1. Flushed skin with itching or burning 2. Difficulty speaking due to laryngeal edema and bronchospasm 3. Tightness in the chest 4. Dyspnea (difficulty/labored breathing) 5. Wheezing 6. Chest pain 7. Hypotension 8. Nausea and vomiting 9. Dizziness 10. Syncope (transient loss of consciousness) 11. Coma

Table 11-2

Diabetic Emergencies[1-3,5-7,15]

Condition	Mechanism and General Information	Possible Signs/Symptoms
Insulin shock	1. Hypoglycemia, which is caused by one or more of the following: • Unpredictable increased amount of glucose used during exercise • Unpredictable increased insulin efficiency with exercise • Not eating enough before exercise or using too much pre-exercise insulin 2. Develops rapidly 3. If prolonged, hypoglycemia can lead to brain injury 4. Pregame anxiety can mimic hypoglycemia 5. Hypoglycemia occurs more often with evening exercise 6. Treated by giving the athlete a sugar substance. Activate EMS if the athlete continues to deteriorate or if there is no improvement in status 30 minutes after sugar ingestion	1. Mental status changes, such as restlessness, impatience, combativeness, and/or bizarre behaviors 2. Diplopia (double vision) 3. Fatigue, weakness, and possibly poor muscle coordination 4. Excessive hunger 5. Occasional tachycardia (usually not present) 6. Nervousness 7. Headache 8. Numbness 9. Palpitations 10. Slurred speech 11. Diaphoresis (excessive sweating) 12. Tremor seizure
Diabetic coma	1. Hyperglycemia, which can be caused by a sudden decrease in regular exercise volume without increasing insulin intake or due to decreased food intake. An infection can also cause an imbalance in the glucose/insulin system 2. Develops slowly over days 3. As the level of glucose in the cells decreases, the cells use other forms of energy, which lead to the production of ketones and organic acids. This leads to the development of ketoacidosis, which can lead to brain damage and death 4. Treatment: • Activate EMS • Give insulin, fluid, and electrolytes	Hyperglycemia: 1. Increased thirst due to dehydration (from glucose spilling into urine) 2. Polyurea (increased urine output over a period of time) 3. Warm and dry skin Ketoacidosis: 1. Abdominal pain 2. Dehydration 3. Restlessness 4. Fruity breath 5. Nausea and vomiting 6. Tachycardia 7. Hypotension 8. Deep respiration/air hunger (Kussmaul's respiration) 9. Decreased level of consciousness

Table 11-3

Common Causes of Nontraumatic Chest Pain[8-11,16,17]

Condition	Mechanism and General Information	Possible Signs/Symptoms
Cardiac		
1. Myocardial infarction (MI)	1. Decreased cardiac perfusion leading to cardiac muscle injury and contractile dysfunction 2. Check for the presence of risk factors, including smoking, diabetes, hypertension, elevated cholesterol level, family history of an early MI, age (men over 40 or postmenopausal women)	1. Heavy tightness and squeezing sensation in the chest 2. Substernal or epigastric pain 3. Radiating pain to the shoulder, jaw, and/or posterior teeth 4. Dyspnea (possibly due to pulmonary edema from MI) 5. Rales or wheezes (pulmonary edema) 6. Skin is flushed, cool, and perspiring 7. Nausea and vomiting 8. Jugular vein distention (see Chapter 1)
2. Hypertrophic cardiomyopathy	A congenital disease causing hypertrophy of the left ventricle, which can cause cardiac blood flow abnormalities and/or impair cardiac function	1. Usually asymptomatic. The first sign may be collapse with sudden death 2. Vague chest pain 3. Dizziness 4. Syncope
3. Mitral valve prolapse	A congenital problem in which the valve between the left atria and ventricle collapses backward during contraction	1. Substernal or left anterior chest pain 2. The pain is usually sharp, lasting minutes or hours 3. Palpitations 4. Usually not exertional 5. Rarely, syncope may occur
4. Marfan's syndrome	1. Congenital problem that can cause connective tissue weakness, which can lead to a dilation or aneurysm of the aorta, as well as many other problems 2. These athletes are usually tall with long arms and fingers. Their arm span may be greater than their height. They also have increased flexibility, an anterior chest wall abnormality, and kyphoscoliosis	Variable
5. Pericarditis	Inflammation of the pericardium (the covering of the heart)	1. Chest pain, radiating to the left arm and upper trapezius 2. Increased pain with coughing, deep breathing, or when in the supine position 3. Dyspnea 4. Nonproductive cough 5. Fever and chills 6. Tachycardia
6. Myocarditis	Inflammation of the heart muscle	1. Recent flu symptoms 2. Dyspnea with exertion 3. Palpitations (sensation of a "skipped beat") 4. Lightheaded

Table 11-3, continued

Condition	Mechanism and General Information	Possible Signs/Symptoms
7. Drug related	Drug use, such as cocaine, anabolic steroids, or amphetamines (speed) may cause cardiac abnormalities	Variable
8. Other congenital causes	Cardiac arrythmias, anomalous coronary arteries, etc	1. Syncope (transient loss of consciousness) 2. Dyspnea 3. Angina (burning chest pain, usually radiating to the left arm) 4. Palpitations
Musculoskeletal Causes		
1. Overuse or degenerative	Overuse or degenerative changes can cause thoracic muscle strains, stress fractures of the ribs, costochondritis, and/or shoulder bursitis and tendonitis	Variable
2. Thoracic spine disorders	This includes a herniated nucleus pulposus, muscle strains, and/or facet joint dysfunctions	1. The pain is usually over the posterior thoracic region 2. There can be anterior chest pain with inspiration, especially in the presence of a facet joint dysfunction
Gastrointestinal Causes		
1. Gastroesophageal reflux	1. This is caused by acid reflux from the stomach into the esophagus 2. Can be due to a hiatal hernia, dysfunction of the lower esophageal sphincter, or other problems that interfere with gastroesophageal motility 3. Increased incidence with exercise	1. Retrosternal burning pain 2. Angina-like chest pain 3. Nonradiating 4. Sour liquid in pharynx 5. Increased pain with eating or laying supine
2. Esophageal spasm	A neuromuscular disorder causing spasms of the esophagus	1. Increased pain with eating and at night 2. Possible dysphagia (difficulty swallowing) 3. Usually not exertional
3. Peptic ulcer	Caused by an ulceration of the mucosal lining of the stomach	1. Burning pain 2. Pain can be in the chest and/or epigastric region 3. Decreased pain with food intake 4. Increased pain at night 5. Pain with palpation of the epigastric region (below the sternum)
4. Gall bladder disease	Can be caused by several factors	1. Dyspepsia 2. Right upper quadrant pain
5. Pancreatis	Inflammation of the pancreas, which can be caused by several reasons	1. Boaring or burning pain 2. Symptoms can mimic a myocardial infarct (MI) 3. Left upper quadrant pain and tenderness

Table 11-3, continued

Condition	Mechanism and General Information	Possible Signs/Symptoms
6. Liver abscess	A localized collection of pus in the liver	1. Pleuritic chest pain (lateral chest pain with muscle splinting and guarding, especially with deep inspirations)
		2. Right upper quadrant pain and tenderness
		3. Fever and chills
		4. Nausea and vomiting
		See Table 11-4
Pulmonary Causes	This includes: asthma, exercised-induced bronchospasm, pneumonia, bronchitis, spontaneous pneumothorax, pleurisy, and pulmonary embolus. See Table 11-4.	
Psychogenic Causes	Anxiety with possible hyperventilation, panic disorder, depression, or a recent psychological stress (including the recent family history of someone having chest pain due to a severe cause) can be underlying factors	1. Recurrent chest pain
		2. Dizziness
		3. Dyspnea
		4. Palpitations
		5. Sweating
		6. Choking
		7. Numbness
		8. Abdominal pain

Table 11-4

Common Causes of Nontraumatic Dyspnea[2,12,17-20]

Condition	Mechanism and General Information	Possible Signs/Symptoms
Airway Obstruction		See Chapter 1
1. Foreign body	Caused by the aspiration of a foreign body	See Tables 11-1 and 11-5
2. Allergic reaction	1. An adverse immune reaction including asthma, anaphylaxis, urticaria, angioedema, and rhinitis (see Anaphylactic Shock in Table 11-1 and Table 11-5)	
3. Respiratory infection	2. This causes airway obstruction due to swelling and/or spasm The most common causes are the common cold, influenza, or bronchitis	1. Cold and influenza: nasal mucous discharge, fever, chills, soar throat, malaise, myalgia, stomach distress
		2. Bronchitis: hacking that produces phlegm cough, malaise, fever, chest wall pain, possible wheezing due to secretions
4. Asthma	1. An allergic reaction that causes the airway to be obstructed due to bronchospasm, inflammation, and excessive bronchial secretions	1. Coughing, which may be a dry cough or a mucous-producing cough
	2. Expiration is more affected than inspiration	2. Shortness of breath
	3. A viral infection, pollens, certain medications, animal danders, molds, odors of fumes, certain foods, dust, or severe psychological emotions can trigger asthma	3. Expanding chest diameter due to limited expiration
		4. Possible wheezing, especially during expiration

Table 11-4, continued

Condition	Mechanism and General Information	Possible Signs/Symptoms
	4. There is usually a personal or family history of asthma in athletes who are having an asthma attack **5.** Treatment: • Have the athlete take puffs of his or her prescribed inhaler (usually one puff every 20 minutes for 2 hours) • Activate EMS if there is cyanosis, exhaustion, difficulty speaking, diaphoresis, and/or decreased mental status	
Diffuse Lung Dysfunction 1. Pneumonia	A bacterial or viral infection of lung tissue	1. Chest pain 2. Fever 3. Productive cough 4. Chills 5. Malaise
2. Spontaneous pneumothorax	See Chapter 8	See Chapter 8
3. Pleurisy	A nonspecific inflammation of the lung lining, usually due to a viral blood infection	1. Severe sharp pain 2. Splinting and muscle guarding with inspiration
Pulmonary Embolism	1. A dislodged clot that enters the lung 2. This can be due to a prolonged period of immobilization, use of oral contraceptives, or after trauma or surgery (especially to the lower extremities) 3. The athlete may have a history of developing deep vein thrombosis	1. Severe pleuretic chest pain (see Pleurisy) 2. Tachycardia 3. Shortness of breath
Cardiogenic	See Table 11-3	See Table 11-3
Psychogenic	See Table 11-3	See Table 11-3
Pulmonary Edema	1. Caused by an accumulation of fluid in the lung tissues and air spaces 2. This can be caused by many conditions, including cardiogenic, drug overdose, exposure to high altitude, central nervous system (CNS) disorders, infections, and other systemic disorders 3. This is very rare in athletes	1. Initial tachypnea, progressing to dyspnea 2. Rales or wheezes with breathing 3. Diaphoresis 4. Apprehension 5. Frothy and bloodstained sputum
Anemia	1. An iron deficiency that leads to low serum ferritin and hemoglobin concentrations 2. Anemia is somewhat common in athletes, especially females. Inadequate iron intake, menstrual loss, gastrointestinal loss, impaired absorption, urinary loss, and sweat loss can cause anemia 3. Anemia is a slow process that is usually asymptomatic until it becomes quite severe	1. Undue exercise fatigue 2. Muscle burning 3. Nausea 4. Pallor (paleness) 5. Pica (compulsive eating of non-nutritional substances) 6. Cheilosis (chapping and fissuring of the lips) 7. Glossitis (inflammation of the tongue)

Table 11-5

Exercise-Induced Allergies[15,19,21-27]

Condition	Mechanism and General Information	Possible Signs/Symptoms
Exercise-induced bronchospasm (EIB)	1. The mechanism of injury is not clear, but it is probably related to airway cooling and water loss 2. EIB is considered a variant of asthma. Therefore, asthmatics have an increased risk for EIB. However, EIB can occur in athletes without a history of asthma 3. EIB develops after 5 to 10 minutes of moderately intense exercise or after stopping exercise. The symptoms plateau, and then usually decrease after 20 to 60 minutes. Some athletes develop another bout of EIB 4 to 12 hours after exercise 4. Factors that can increase the risk of developing EIB include air pollution, exercising in dry cold air, increased ozone, pollens, and certain foods (shrimp, celery, peanuts, egg whites, almonds, and bananas) 5. EIB affects up to 15% of the population	1. Dsypnea 2. Coughing 3. Tachycardia 4. Wheezing 5. Fatigue and prolonged postexercise recovery time 6. Prolonged expiration phase of breathing 7. Contraction of accessory breathing muscles 8. Hypertension 9. Burning in chest 10. Anxiety 11. Soar throat 12. Headache 13. Stomach cramps or nausea
Exercise-induced Urticaria	1. The development of small pruritic papular wheals that occur during of after exercise 2. The exact mechanism is unknown, but it is related to exposure to heat, fever, hot showers, and anxiety	1. The rash starts on the trunk and neck before spreading to the rest of the body 2. Bronchospasm may occur
Exercise-induced anaphylaxis	1. An anaphylactic reaction due to high-intensity exercise 2. See Anaphylactic Shock in Table 11-1 3. It does not occur with every exercise bout 4. The exact cause is unknown 5. The risk factors include a positive personal or family history of the problem, exercise in hot humid weather, pollens, certain medications, and eating certain foods prior to exercise (see listing in EIB section) 6. The symptoms may start 5 minutes into exercise and last up to 4 hours after exercise 7. The athlete can have a mild reaction, such as itching or a full-blown case of anaphylactic shock	1. Pruritus (itching) 2. Large urticaria wheals (localized edema and dilation) 3. Angioedema (subcutaneous edema due to dilation and increased permeability of the capillaries) affecting the face, extremities, and oral cavity 4. Flushing of skin 5. Dyspnea due to an upper airway obstruction 6. Headache 7. Stridor (harsh wheeze) with breathing and possible choking 8. Syncope 9. Nausea and vomiting 10. Hypotension

Table 11-6

Common Nontraumatic Abdominal Disorders[2,15,28,29]

Condition	Mechanism and General Information	Possible Signs/Symptoms
Esophageal reflux	See section on Esophageal Reflux	
Peptic ulcer	See section on Peptic Ulcer	
Irritable bowel syndrome	1. Altered bowel habits without any organic disease 2. Possible causes include an alteration in motility or reflexes, carbohydrate intolerance, or psychological stress	1. Abdominal pain 2. Bloating
Diarrhea	1. A frequent and watery unformed stool 2. Can be caused by exercise, an infectious disease, Crohn's disease, ulcerative colitis, and many other possibilities	1. Watery bowel movements 2. Cramping 3. Urgency
Dyspepsia	1. A collective term to describe upper gastrointestinal GI complaints 2. Some of the conditions it describes include gastric reflux, peptic ulcer disease, general indigestion (perhaps due to a nervous athlete), effects of nonsteroidal anti-inflammatory and antibiotic drugs, caffeine ingestion, and others	1. Abdominal pain 2. Nausea 3. Heartburn 4. Indigestion
Constipation	1. Decreased frequency of bowel movements or difficulty evacuating a bowel movement. Defecation may be delayed for days or the stool may be hard 2. This can be caused by several diseases and dysfunction's of the lower GI tract, low fiber in the diet, or anxiety	1. Decreased frequency of feces evacuation 2. Difficulty with feces evacuation
Gastroenteritis	1. Inflammation of the upper GI tract, usually due to an infection	1. Stomach pain 2. Nausea and vomiting 3. Diarrhea 4. Fever and myalgia
Gastritis	1. Inflammation of the mucosal lining in the stomach 2. This can be caused by medications, stress, or alcohol	1. Pain in the left upper quadrant or epigastric region
Hemorrhoids	1. A varicosity of the veins that are internal or external to the anus 2. Can be caused by the valsalva maneuver	1. Anal bleeding 2. Itching
Sickle cell anemia	1. A genetic structural defect in the hemoglobin molecule that occurs primarily in African-American people 2. Athletes with this condition can develop an acute syndrome that manifests itself with severe pain. This is a medical emergency	Acute syndrome: 1. Possible acute abdominal and chest pain 2. Severe skeletal pain 3. Fever 4. Jaundice

Table 11-7

Common Nontraumatic Exercise-Induced Abdominal Disorders[15,18]

Condition	Mechanism and General Information
Exercise-Induced Abdominal Disorders	
1. Upper GI motility disorders	Heartburn and nausea that can occur due to slower gastric emptying times with moderate to intense exercise. Also, there is an increase of gastric reflux with exercise due to increased air swallowing and relaxation of the lower esophageal sphincter.
2. Lower GI mobility disorders	Cramping, urgency, and/or diarrhea that can be due to an increased gut motility from the mechanical pounding of running and bouncing, a massaging effect of the psoas contracting against the intestine, and/or autonomic nervous system changes. These symptoms can also be due to decreased blood flow and ischemia of the intestine that can occur during moderate to intense exercise.
3. GI bleeding	Rectal bleeding, thought to be due to decreased blood flow and ischemia of the intestinal tract that occurs during moderate to intense exercise.
4. Hematuria	Blood in the urine, thought to be due to a rupture of renal capillaries or an empty bladder flipping up and down during running and bouncing.

References

1. Bledsoe B, Porter R, Shade B. Brady *Paramedic Emergency Care. 3rd ed.* Upper Saddle River, NJ: Brady Prentice Hall;1997:303-329,469-497,553-569,725-737,776-782.
2. Booher J, Thibodeau G. *Athletic Injury Assessment. 3rd ed.* St. Louis, Mo: Mosby;1994:128-130,354-395.
3. Voight M. Emergency care and on-the-field management. In: Sanders B, ed. *Sports Physical Therapy.* Norwalk, Conn: Appleton & Lange;1990:45-59.
4. Kinzer KW. Treating insect stings. *Phys Sporstmed.* 1991;19(8):33-36.
5. Taunton JE, McCargar L. Managing activity in patients who have diabetes. *Phys Sportsmed.* 1995;23(3):41-52.
6. Robbins DC, Charleton S. Managing the diabetic athlete. *Phys Sportsmed.* 1989;17(12):45-54.
7. Berg K. The diabetic athlete. In: Mellion MB, Walsh WM, Shelton GL, eds. *The Team Physician's Handbook.* Philadelphia, Pa: Hanley & Belfus; 1990:189-193.
8. Billups D, Martin D, Swain RA. Training room evaluation of chest pain in the adolescent athlete. *South Med J.* 1995;88:667-672.
9. Cishek MB, Moser KM, Amsterdam EA. Chest pain: working up nonemergent conditions. *J Resp Diseases.* 1996;17:560-572.
10. Bernhardt DT, Landry GL. Chest pain in active young people. *Phys Sportsmed.* 1994;22(6):70-85.
11. Cheitlin MD. Evaluating athletes who have heart symptoms. *Phys Sportsmed.* 1993;21(3):150-162.
12. Marino N, Bruno P. Cardiopulmonary conditions. In: Scuderi G, McCann P, Bruno P, eds. *Sports Medicine: Principles of Primary Care.* St. Louis, Mo: Mosby; 1996:18-34.
13. Putukian M. Don't miss gastrointestinal disorders in athletes. *Phys Sportsmed.* 1997;25(11):80-94.
14. Bergman RT. Assessing acute abdominal pain. *Phys Sportsmed.* 1996;24(4):72-82.
15. Dreibelbeis MJ. Nonorthopedic problems. In: Sanders B, ed. *Sports Physical Therapy.* Norwalk, Conn: Appleton & Lange; 1990:273-287.
16. Henderson JM. Ruling out danger: differential diagnosis of thoracic pain. *Phys Sportsmed.* 1992;20(9):124-132.
17. Rund DA. Emergency evaluation of chest pain. *Phys Sportsmed.* 1990;18(4):69-72.
18. Harris SS. Helping active women avoid anemia. *Phys Sportsmed.* 1995;23(5):35-46.
19. Rund DA. Asthma. *Phys Sportsmed.* 1990;18(1):143-146.
20. Sitorius MA, Mellion MB. General medical problems. In: Mellion MB, Walsh WM, Shelton GL, eds. *The Team Physician's Handbook.* Philadelphia, Pa: Hanley & Belfus; 1990:161-178.
21. Blumenthal MN. Sports-aggravated allergies. *Phys Sportsmed.* 1990;18(12):52-66.
22. Hutchens, M. Exercise-induced allergic reactions. In: Andrews JR, Clancy WG, Whiteside JA, eds. *On-Field Evaluation and Treatment of Common Athletic Injuries.* St. Louis, Mo: Mosby; 1997:30-36.
23. Mahler DA. Exercise-induced asthma. *Med Sci Sports Exer.* 1993;25:554-561.
24. Rupp NT. Diagnosis and management of exercise-induced asthma. *Phys Sportsmed.* 1996;24(1):77-87.
25. Storms WW, Joyner DM. Update on exercise-induced-asthma. *Phys Sportsmed.* 1997;25(3):45-55.
26. TerrellT, Hough DO, Alexander R. Identifying exercise allergies. *Phys Sportsmed.* 1996;24(11):76-89.
27. Wise SL, Stafford CT. Anaphylaxis from exercise. *Emer Med.* 1991;June 15:141-144.
28. Cohen SA, Siegel JH. Gastrointestinal system. In: Scuderi GR, McCann PD, Bruno PJ, eds. *Sports Medicine: Principles of Primary Care.* St. Louis, Mo: Mosby; 1997:39-45.

29. Mellman MF, Podesta L. Common medical problems in sports. *Clin Sports Med.* 1997;16:635-662.
30. Green GA. Exercise-induced gastrointestinal symptoms. *Phys Sportsmed.* 1993;21(10):60-70.

Bibliography

Adelman DC, Spector SL. Acute respiratory emergencies in emergency treatment of the injured athlete. *Clin Sports Med.* 1989;8:71-78.

Agonstini R. Women in sports. In: Mellion MB, Walsh WM, Shelton GL, eds. *The Team Physician's Handbook.* Philadelphia, Pa: Hanley & Belfus; 1990:179-188.

Lambert SD. Environmental conditions. In: Sanders B, ed. *Sports Physical Therapy.* Norwalk, Conn: Appleton & Lange; 1990:61-78.

Mellion MB, Shelton GL. Safe exercise in the heat and heat injuries. In: Mellion MB, Walsh WM, Shelton GL, eds. *The Team Physician's Handbook.* Philadelphia, Pa: Hanley & Belfus; 1990:59-69.

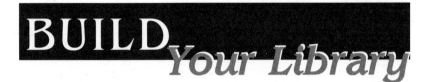

BUILD Your Library

This book and many others on numerous different topics are available from SLACK Incorporated. For further information or a copy of our latest catalog, contact us at:

Professional Book Division
SLACK Incorporated
6900 Grove Road
Thorofare, NJ 08086 USA
Telephone: 1-856-848-1000
1-800-257-8290
Fax: 1-856-853-5991
E-mail: orders@slackinc.com
www.slackinc.com

We accept most major credit cards and checks or money orders in US dollars drawn on a US bank. Most orders are shipped within 72 hours.

Contact us for information on recent releases, forthcoming titles, and bestsellers. If you have a comment about this title or see a need for a new book, direct your correspondence to the Editorial Director at the above address.

Thank you for your interest and we hope you found this work beneficial.